THE CANKER SORE CURE

How To Eliminate Mouth Ulcers Naturally
And Improve Health Exponentially

Patrick McCleary

www.cankersorecure.com

Table of Contents

CHAPTER 1

My Story

"The greater the obstacle, the more glory in overcoming it."
– Molière

My first, lovely rendezvous with mouth sores (aka canker sores, mouth ulcers, aphthous ulcers or aphthous stomatitis) occurred when I had had a very bad reaction to an antibiotic. When I was in my 30s, I was experiencing severe chronic sinus infections that would seem to get better and then within weeks would reoccur. This happened over and over again for over a year before I figured out the reason why. During this time, my doctor was having me try different antibiotics which were only working on a temporary basis. It was very frustrating. After fifteen months of this, an ENT specialist had me get X-rays of my sinuses. The results showed that I had cysts in my maxillary sinus cavities. I subsequently had sinus surgery to remove them. This took care of the chronic infections.

During the time that I was taking the various medications, I was prescribed a sulfa-based antibiotic. After taking it for a few days, I started having severe headaches. If you've ever had a sinus infection, you know that headaches are a very common side effect. I kept taking the antibiotic thinking that the headaches were related to the sinus infection. A few days later, things regressed. I developed a high fever; I then became lethargic and the inside of my mouth broke out with mouth sores everywhere - and I mean everywhere. Not only this, I also got sores at the other end of the digestive tract. You're probably familiar with this area as you deal with it on a daily basis. I don't want to gross you out with too much detail here. Let's just say I had these sores "coming and going!"

These mouth sores were so bad and painful that I could not eat solid food. I could only drink smoothies with a straw. The ones on the "exit" side were just as bad. Imagine the fun I had pooping. Needless to say, both my wife and I were very concerned. I went back to see my doctor and he ordered blood work on me. The results showed that my white blood cell count had dropped to "high alarm" levels. White blood cells are the "immune cells" that protect the body from infection and foreign invaders. A little research at the time showed that cancer patients typically had similar low white blood cell counts to what I was experiencing. I was more miserable than you can imagine. I felt like a zombie. I was very scared and I was starting to wonder if I was getting close to the end of the road for my life.

After a week of this illness, I decided to visit with a hematologist to see what he could uncover about my situation. In the meantime, I was put on some very powerful antibiotics and steroids even though my doctor was not sure of what was happening with me. This particular hematologist was a very thoughtful fellow and he asked me all kinds of questions. He was wanting to pinpoint everything I was doing within the sequence of events that led me to where I was at that moment. I am grateful for this because he took everything in and was able to deduce that I might have had an allergic reaction to the antibiotic. For the first time, I felt a little emotional relief and hope.

It turns out he was right. I am highly allergic to sulfa-based antibiotics. Thus, the beginning of my adventure with years of chronic mouth sores that got worse over time. One thing I learned from that experience is that mouth sores thrive in a body with a weak immune system. This is one of the many triggers. In the next chapter, we'll discuss these triggers in more detail. For now, bear with me while I share a little bit more of my experiences with these "fun" little guys.

After my sinuses were healed, whenever I would begin to feel run down, I would typically get cold sores on my lips more so than mouth sores. But things started to change in my 40s. It was during this time that the cold sores lessened while I started to experience an increase of mouth sores. Before continuing with my progression in time, let me share some insights about me. As an adult, I've always been very health conscious. I exercise a lot, I meditate, and we've always eaten what we consider healthy foods. Striving for good health will always be very important to me. Even though I considered myself to be leading a healthy lifestyle, I was still having to deal with these nasty mouth sores on occasion. Perhaps you've had similar experiences to mine with mouth sores or other health issues.

I seemed to get these sores at the worst possible times like at Christmas or while on vacations. Ugh! Nothing I purchased at the drug store seemed to alleviate them. I tried everything you can possibly imagine. I was desperate for relief and a solution to this chronic problem. Eventually, when I would get an outbreak, I would visit my primary physician and they would prescribe prednisone. This medicine is a steroid and too much of it over time can cause harmful effects in the body such as weakening of the bones. I wasn't too concerned about this because it dramatically sped up the healing time from a breakout of mouth sores. Unfortunately, over time, the reoccurrence of mouth sores was exceeding the Prednisone limit from my physician. Knowing that I could not get the Prednisone prescription as often as I wanted, I took the matter in my own hands and ordered some from Canada. You can get a lot of medicine from Canada without a prescription. I'm sad to say that my suffering outweighed my concern about the long-term negative effects this medicine might be doing to me. This is partly why I'm sharing my story. I don't want you to have to go through what I went through and that's what motivated me to write this book.

An interesting irony is that over the years I became more health conscious and yet the reoccurrence of mouth sores increased. I was growing more and more frustrated with all of this. I was very healthy in every respect with the exception of experiencing mouth sores. It got to the point where it became chronic. I started experiencing them on a monthly basis. I guess the blessing here is that it really motivated me to continue to work towards solving this miserable puzzle.

If you're reading this book, you probably don't need me to tell you how painful mouth sores can be. You wouldn't think that a tiny little spot in your mouth the size of pin head could cause much pain. But boy oh boy are they painful, particularly when you have to eat something. I would typically get more than one at a time too. I spent hours and hours researching online how to heal them and I would try everything and anything to heal and prevent them but, to no avail, I kept getting outbreaks of them.

Mouth sores kind of fall into that "never never land" where the medical profession cannot seem to pinpoint what causes them or how to eliminate them. They know some things like food allergies and spicy foods might trigger them and yet people would eliminate some these things and they would still experience them. That's what happened with me. Every time I went to see my doctor, I would hear something like, "here, try this and this and hopefully it will help but that's all we can do for you at this time." Well, that was not going to cut for me. I was determined to get to the bottom of it and eliminate mouth sores from my life for good.

An interesting statistic that I discovered is that over half the population of the world will experience oral mouth sores during some point in their life. That's a lot people! You would think that the medical profession would have Mouth Sore Specialists with that many people having to deal with them. Have you heard the term, "no pain, no gain?" Well, I had had enough pain and I certainly wasn't gaining anything. The constant reoccurrence of mouth sores turned out to be a blessing. It gave me the motivation for me to figure out a cure for once and for all. To be honest, at the time I was thinking I would be really happy if I could just reduce the occurrence of them.

Take heart as I'm about to share with you everything that I've done to eradicate them from my life. If you're reading this book and you've stuck with me this far, then you're likely very motivated to solve this problem. Now, I cannot say emphatically that I will never get a mouth sore again. There's always the possibility of something else popping up in my life experience that triggers one. However, knowing what I know now, if this does happen, I'll have the confidence to figure out the cause fairly quickly and eliminate that source for good.

I'm happy to say that I haven't had a mouth sore for a very long time, and I want my blessing to be your blessing. I would like to be your guide and source of encouragement over the coming chapters to help you eliminate these irritants from your life. All you need to do is follow the protocol as outlined in this book. I promise this process will not cause you anything close to the discomfort you experience when you get a breakout of mouth sores. Not only will you greatly reduce or eliminate these annoying mouth sores, you'll also get to experience a wonderful byproduct, which to me is as good if not better: you will also be substantially improving your overall health, you'll have more energy and you'll be able to make the most out of your life and future. If you don't have your health, it's really hard to enjoy life. There's a saying, "health is wealth." I have certainly found this to be true in my life. I've been one who has invested a lot of time and effort into creating optimal health, not only for the present time, but also for the later years. I know everything I do on a daily basis is also an investment, good or bad, for my golden years. I do want them to be golden. I desire to live fully now and in the future. This is why I have placed so much emphasis on my health and fitness.

Before we can get into this process of eliminating our mouth sores and improving our overall health, it is important to learn what causes them in the first place.

CHAPTER 2

Causes of Mouth Sores

"As long as you keep searching, the answers will come."
- Joan Baez

In my research to uncover what causes these painful mouth sores, it became clear that there is not one clear cut answer. It took a lot of digging and paying attention to my own personal experiences with them to gain valuable insights about them. I'm not a doctor or a certified health professional, however, I am an expert at dealing with mouth sores. Believe me, it was a not a personal calling or a desire to be an expert at this. I never thought I would write a book about it, that's for sure. If this book can alleviate some of the suffering that I've experienced over many years for you or anyone that reads this book, then it will be well worth it to have put these words on paper.

I believe that one thing we can likely agree on is that there are many causes and triggers for mouth sores. A major cause of mouth sores is often referred to as an *immune deficiency disorder*. There are basically two type of immune deficiency disorders. The first is a weak (low activity) immune system and the second is an autoimmune (high activity) disorder. With a weak immune system, your body cannot do enough on its own to keep you in optimal health and fight off infections and sickness. With an autoimmune deficiency disorder, your immune system is basically in overdrive. It's fighting fires but having a hard time keeping up with all of them. Here's a good analogy: Think of a teacup. You have this nice teacup and you start to pour hot water into it. When the water gets to the top, you keep pouring. What happens? It runs down the side of the teacup, then it runs all over the table and onto the floor, and then you have this nice mess to clean up. Now, think of your body like the teacup. When we keep pouring into our body the wrong things and don't stop, eventually our body can't handle it any longer and starts to break down. We then experience illness and *dis-ease*.

A weak immune system can cause mouth sores by itself or get supercharged in combination with other causes and triggers that I'll soon share with you. When the "supercharged" effect happens, watch out! This is where you can experience a breakout of multiple mouth sores. Nothing is more frustrating than trying to keep these suckers under control, hoping the worst is over and then, before you know it, a couple more pop up in your mouth. If you cannot handle a lot of pain, you definitely don't want to be on the "multiple mouth sores" train. You'll be wanting to jump off before you can say "choo choo."

Poor health equates to increased odds of immune deficiency disorders. As you read this book, you'll be learning a number of simple and effective ways to boost your immune system and improve your health. This is the secret to the long-term solution of reducing them or eliminating them altogether. When you strengthen the immune system, you start to minimize the effects of getting mouth sores from the various causes and triggers. Getting back to my analogy, it would be like transforming the teacup into a tea pot. You can pour a lot more water into a pot rather than a cup before it starts to overflow.

The decisions and choices we make with regards to our diet, exercise, living environment, and so on can significantly impact our immune system. However, what if there was also another underlying cause of mouth sores that we have nothing to do with? What if there is something else lurking in our bodies and wreaking havoc with our immune system and it's not our fault.

I am going to be talking about this underlying cause in Chapter 6 when we discuss diet. The reason for doing this is because your diet is the key to eliminating this underlying cause. If you can't wait until Chapter 6 to find out, feel free to glance ahead at this chapter to satisfy your curiosity and then come back here to pick up where you left off.

Now that you understand a little bit about how health of your immune system affects the frequency (or lack thereof) of mouth sores, let's move on to the next cause. A major contributor to mouth sores is an allergy-like reaction to certain foods. These foods might not normally trigger mouth sores in a completely healthy body. However, if there is something else going on in your body that is causing your immune system to be in overdrive, certain foods have been shown to trigger a breakout of mouth sores. As you strengthen your immune system and improve your overall health, you should be able to reintroduce back into your diet some of these trigger foods, many of which are really good for you.

Let's start with what I believe to be the grandaddy of them all and the top food-related cause for mouth sores: spicy foods. I've never been a fan of spicy foods but would eat some spicy food on occasion, mainly when I did not know that the food I was being served was spicy. This is because I might be at a friend's house for dinner or dining at a restaurant. Have you ever asked a server if a certain dish is hot or spicy and be told it was not, only to find out that it was incredibly spicy? This has happened to me many times. Everyone's tolerance for spicy foods is different. In this situation, the server likely loves spicy foods and a dish with very little spice to it is, for them, considered not spicy at all.

I learned the hard way how spicy foods can be the impetus for mouth sores. I remember the day very clearly. It was a Saturday night and we had gotten some carryout burritos. Sometimes, on the weekends, we like to get some carryout and watch a good movie. On this occasion, I was particularly hungry. Unfortunately for me, the burritos were very spicy. My hunger and this spicy burrito in front of me was the worst possible combination. I decided to just eat it and enjoy it. It was hot to say the least. I remember thinking to myself, *"well, my mouth is already on fire so just finish it."* When I finished it, my entire inside of mouth was red. I was having a major allergic reaction to the spices in the food. Take a guess as to what happened next. The mouth sores started popping out one by one, growing like weeds in my entire mouth. They were everywhere. It was one of the most miserable experiences I ever had with them. I went to my doctor and she looked inside my mouth, squinted her eyes and gave that "you poor soul" look all over her face. She prescribed Prednisone to help them clear up faster. As these outbreaks started occurring more frequently, I got accustomed to asking my doctor for Prednisone. Sometimes I had to beg because my doctor was concerned about giving me too much as overtaking it can cause bone loss and other health issues.

I would like to clarify something here before we go further. I'm not saying that every person prone to mouth sores who eats spicy foods is going to get an outbreak of them. Our bodies are different. Keep that in mind as you read this book. You are going to want to learn the hot buttons that give you an outbreak. The information you're about to learn will show you what might be the common denominators for you. You are going to learn to pay attention to what you eat and to eliminate the likely causes and triggers. When going through this process of elimination, it is better to err on the safe side. In the future, once you have your mouth health under control, you should be able to reintroduce some of these foods back into your diet. I know for me it's very simple. Personally, I was not interested in taking a chance on certain foods that I knew caused an issue for me in the past. As you will see, I did everything in my power to not ever experience one mouth sore again. I want to encourage you be willing to do whatever it takes to eliminate these irritating mouth sores from your life. If I can do it, then so can you.

Let's move on to the next cause. This also has to do with the foods you eat. Most foods are either acidic or alkaline in nature. There are some foods that are neutral, however, for the sake of this explanation, we're only going to be discussing acidity and alkalinity. The unit of measurement for the level of acidity or alkalinity in food is the pH number (power of Hydrogen.) An example would be using a range of numbers from 0 to 14. Pertaining to a specific food, the lower the number, the more acidic it is and, the higher the number, the more alkaline it is. The number 7 typically means neutral and any number below 7 means acidic, with 0 being the most acidic. Any number above 7 means alkaline with 14 being the most alkaline. A simple search online will give you a food chart showing the pH level for most foods.

Your diet plays such a critical role in the reduction or elimination of mouth sores. Chapter 6 will be all about diet and you'll be learning the importance of eating more healthy, alkaline foods. These foods will help boost your immune system and get you on the road to a healthy lifestyle. Over many generations of our human ancestral history, we moved from eating a healthy, alkaline diet to an unhealthy, acidic diet. Our ancestors ate mostly fresh, organic and unprocessed foods. They ate what was in season and lived off the land. Today, we eat a lot of processed foods containing chemicals and preservatives and we've become addicted to sugar and unhealthy fats. If you want to get rid of those painful sores in your mouth, you're going to have to participate in our little "health club" and eat less acidic foods and more alkaline foods. Hey, think about it for a minute. Is it so bad that you have to eat healthier foods to not have to experience severe and lasting pain in your mouth on occasion? Can you also see the potential for some nice side benefits? Do you like the idea of living a long and healthy life and rarely ever getting an illness or disease? If so, I think you'll appreciate many or all of the methods and techniques for mouth sore prevention. The good news is that your purchase of this book entitles you to a lifetime membership to my "health club." However, like with a gym, your membership by itself is not going to make you healthier. You have to get off your duff and do the right things consistently and persistently to see the positive changes in your life. The cool thing is unlike a gym, there are no monthly fees here. All you need to do is read the book and follow the plan. Simple as apple pie. Wait, that's highly acidic, so let me change that to *simple as a bowl of almonds.*

There are some important things to understand as we discuss acidity and alkalinity. The foods that you eat have to hang out in your mouth for a bit as you chew and before working their way to the stomach. Certain acidic foods can trigger a breakout of mouth sores under the right conditions such as a weakened immune system. Acidic foods can also worsen mouth sores and cause them to proliferate. Lemon and limes are a paradox when it comes to mouth sores. They are acidic while inside your mouth, however, once metabolized in your stomach, they become highly alkaline. They are therefore classified as highly alkaline foods with a very high pH number. Although lemons and limes are good for you, if you are dealing with chronic mouth sores, it might be good idea to avoid them for a while.

Some common acidic foods involved with mouth sores are spicy foods, pineapple, citrus fruits, vinegar products, wine and other types of alcohol. We'll talk more about these and other foods in Chapter 4 where we discuss the foods to eliminate from our diet for a period of time. Before you get too upset about having to give up some of your favorite foods, I did say *for a period of time.* You'll be able to reintroduce them later if you wish after you have things under control.

As previously mentioned, we can be allergic to certain foods. My wife and I like to eat a good healthy salad for lunch. One day, my wife used olive oil and red wine vinegar as the salad dressing. I started eating the salad and my tongue and the area underneath started feeling hot and sore. I looked in the mirror and it was very red. Within 30 minutes I broke out with a mouth sore under my tongue. I was amazed at how fast it happened. It didn't take long to figure out that I had an immediate allergic reaction to the red wine vinegar. Some further research on my part showed that certain vinegar products can cause mouth sores. It was an easy decision for me to stop eating all vinegar dressings including balsamic vinegar which I so love. If you recall, I had one goal in mind when I started this journey and that was to completely eliminate the occurrence of mouth sores. I was willing to do whatever it takes to keep them at bay. You'll better understand my reasons why as you read this book. I would love to see you become one of the next fortunate souls who eliminates them from their life experience.

By now you may be thinking that your overall health correlates to the level of occurrences of mouth sores. It does and it doesn't depending on your definition of good health. Let me share more background story to help you see the big picture.

I have always valued good health and fitness. Even as a young adult, I understood that what we do with our bodies will determine our overall quality of life. Being so young, I didn't have to do as much to stay somewhat fit. However, I also intuitively knew that the extra effort I put into my health and fitness would pay off in spades as I grew older. I've wanted to be fit and active my entire life. Although I'm a lot older now than when I was when I first had those ideas, I am still very youthful and fit because I am constantly doing the right things for my body. This is a huge priority for me.

My wife and I have always been into healthy eating, however, our perception of what healthy eating means has changed quite drastically over the years. We've always strived to eat healthy foods for the most part. We purchased organic foods as much as possible. We drank mostly water and tea for our beverage intake. We also subscribed to the notion that eating certain less healthy foods and things like sweets in moderation was okay. We definitely bought into this concept for many years. I'll be honest, one of my favorite foods of all-time has been cheese pizza. I certainly had my fair share of pizza in my life. Also, as I grew older, my sweet quotient seemed to increase. I tease my wife all the time that she transferred some of her sweet tooth to me after we met. To set the record straight once and for all, I'm going to take responsibility for my sweet tooth. I was just a little older before the allure of sweets overcame me. We did pretty well with what we knew at that time about healthy eating. If I compare my current diet with the diets of the past, it is like night and day. It has evolved to being a super healthy and primarily plant-based diet. You'll be learning about this diet and the foods I avoid in the pages ahead.

Exercising has always been very important to me ever since I was a young lad. I typically exercise six or seven days per week. I used to ride my bike for exercise but fell in love with running as a middle-aged adult. These days, I typically run six or seven days per week. I sometimes bike, do the elliptical machine or swim as a way to mix up. Exercise is a wonderful way to boost your immune system. It is definitely something to consider for helping you win the battle with mouth sores. In Chapter 7, we will get into more depth about exercise and the role it plays in a healthy and long-lasting body.

One of the things I'm most passionate about is personal development and self-growth. I've always been curious as to what makes us tick as human beings and how we influence the experiences that we have in our lives on a day to day basis. I'm a truth seeker. I'm about building my inner and outer awareness so that I can make the best possible choices in my life at all times. It's my intention to be *at cause* over my life rather than a victim of my circumstances. This passion led me to become a personal development junkie. I have boxes and boxes of personal development books. I soaked it all in. I came to see that one of the most important things I can do for my overall quality of life experience is to exercise my mind like I exercise my body. In Chapter 9, I'll expand upon these principles to give you a better understanding of how to incorporate personal development into your daily routine.

Over the years my knowledge of healthy eating, exercising and improving my mindset had certainly improved. But in spite of all of these wonderful things that I did for myself, I still got mouth sores - and lots of them. And these mouth sores not only kept showing up, they also became more chronic in nature. Maybe you can relate to this story. After all, if you're reading this book, you're likely experiencing them or some other weird *dis-ease*. It is quite frustrating to consider yourself a very healthy person and, at the same time, be experiencing these painful sores on a frequent basis. However, if it weren't for my suffering and frustration, I would not be where I am today and for that I am very grateful.

I have come to see healthy lifestyle is just one of many potential factors here. I had to dig deeper. I had to do some research and find out what else played a role besides overall striving for good health. I knew this was very important but how do we define "good health?" I was healthy in every respect, hardly ever got sick, and yet I still experienced chronic mouth sores. Was I healthy or not? I guess the answer is that I was somewhat healthy but not healthy enough. I was determined to get to the bottom of it. If we want to define great health in a pure sense, it would seem that it would mean fitness and vigor, a lack of illness, disorder and disease. In that sense, I can't say I was in good health even though apart from the mouth sores, I was in pretty good shape.

The technical name for a mouth or canker sore is Aphthous Stomatitis. It is a benign condition that occurs a number of times per year in an *otherwise healthy individual*. The first thing I thought when I read this definition was, *yep, they're talking about me.* Over 50% of the population will experience mouth sores at some point in their life and the medical field has yet to uncover the underlying cause of them. I guess it hasn't been a priority because they are benign and heal on their own over a period of one to three weeks. Well, their loss is my gain. I figured out the solutions and I am excited to share all of this information with you.

Being that I'm a big-picture guy, when I looked at my overall health, I was obviously not as healthy as I wanted to be. I had to shift gears and decide that I wanted to be in great health, not just good health. Good health was obviously not working for me. I knew I had to find a way to make my overall immune system stronger. I decided great health would mean that the pistons were firing on all cylinders and that I had none or very rare occurrences of sickness, disease and disorders, especially mouth sores. It was time to step up my game. So, let's go back to that earlier thought where I said health does and does not play a role in getting mouth sore. The "does" part is referring to striving for great health. That's where you're going with this book. To create a path for you to experience an extreme, healthy lifestyle along with a very strong immune system. The "does not" part relates to those things outside of being in great health that can cause mouth sores such as allergic reactions to certain foods, underlying viruses and trauma to inner mouth tissue. I am referring to deep-rooted causes that take a more targeted approach to resolve.

I haven't discussed trauma to the inner tissue of the mouth, but I know this to also be a big factor in my own experience. Have you ever bitten the inside of your cheeks accidentally? I have many times and there have been several occasions where a mouth sore would show up right after I bit the inside of my cheek. This is because weak tissue can be fertile grounds for them. There have also been instances reported where brushing your teeth with hard toothbrush bristles can cause some trauma to the gums and lead to mouth sores. Also, toothpaste containing SLS (sodium lauryl sulphate) has been known to cause mouth sores. SLS is a surfactant that is typically used as a cleaning agent and is a known food allergen. As you can see, it's important to make sure that we aren't doing things unintentionally to our mouth which contributes to a breakout of mouth sores.

Another factor that plays a significant role in mouth sores is stress. When we are under duress or stress, it can instantly impact our immune system. It can also impact our digestive system and, guess what, our mouth is part of our digestive system. Ulcers are very common in people who experience a lot of stress. A mouth sore is an ulcer. All of these things are interconnected like a giant spider web. When one thing breaks down, it can cause another thing to break down. Stress affects people in different ways. If you're prone to mouth sores, your *dis-ease* or disorder is going to take the path of least resistance and this is why they occur for you. For other people, stress might trigger things like migraine headaches or skin disorders.

Let's pause to see where we are thus far. We've determined that there are a variety of reasons why we experience mouth sores. There is the foundational issue which is a weak or overactive immune system. In dealing with the immune system, we have to take a long-term approach to making it better. It is not an overnight fix. There are also more immediate triggers such allergic reaction to foods or trauma to the mouth tissue. We will cover all of the issues in the coming chapters with the emphasis on removing toxins and building a strong immune system.

In the next chapter we'll be discussing the game plan for how to deal with mouth sores when you experience them and the many approaches to reduce or eliminate them altogether. So, grab your cup of green tea and let's get this party started.

CHAPTER 3

Gearing Up for the Game Plan

"A strategy, even a great one, doesn't implement itself."
- Jeroen De Flander

In order for you to completely eliminate or drastically reduce the occurrence of mouths sores from your life, you're going to have to attack them from multiple fronts. You will first want to remove those potential triggers that can be dealt with immediately such as allergic reactions and trauma to the mouth. Then you will want to follow my long-term plan for eliminating toxins, strengthening your immune system and creating great health. This two-pronged approach is how I finally eliminated them from my life. The wonderful byproduct of all of this is that I'm healthier than I've ever been and I'm excited about the years ahead. I'm confident that as I grow older, I'll be as young and fit as I can possibly be. Are you excited about the possibility of getting younger as you grow older?

I have previously stated that being healthy and fit as always been a priority of mine. I got a nice confirmation of this when my wife, Nancy, became a certified health coach. She studied under the Dr. William Sears Wellness Institute[1]. Most people understand the importance of investing in retirement accounts such as an IRA

---

[1] **drsearswellnessinstitute.com**

during our working career. This is so when those retirement years finally come around, we have money to cover our expenses and enjoy our golden years. None of us want to face retirement worrying about how to pay the bills or have a good time. Health also plays a very critical role in the quality our retirement years.

Dr. Sears, in his book, *Prime Time Health: A Scientifically Proven Plan for Feeling Younger and Living Longer*, discusses how people save money for retirement but never give much thought to investing in their body to better enjoy it. He further states that most people don't appreciate their health until they lose it. Dr. Sears advises everyone to set up an IRAH, or Individual Retirement Account for Health. This means you right away start to invest more time and money into your health quotient. At I write this, 55% of Americans take prescription drugs on a regular basis. And, according to the health research firm, QuintilesIMS[2], the number of prescriptions filled rose 85% between 1997 and 2016. This is absolutely mind-boggling to me.

People are spending hundreds of dollars extra per month on prescriptions drugs and complaining about it, but they keep doing it because *they believe* they have no other choice. I stress those words "they believe" because they are ignorant that there is a better way or they simply don't care enough about their health to make better choices for themselves. Would you rather be investing a few hundred dollars per month in your IRAH or on pharmaceutical drugs that may ultimately make you worse off in the long run? I want you to take back control of your health and life. I want

---

[2] **iqvia.com (formerly QuintilesIMS), a health-care informatics company**

you to live *the great life*! This all starts with your mindset. We'll discuss mindset in Chapter 9 but I want you to start thinking about your Future Healthy Self right now.

If you'll allow me, I would like to be your mentor and source of encouragement on this short journey while you read this book and make some powerful changes in your life. You are at a turning point right now, as you read these words. What you do from this point further will have a dramatic impact on the quality of the rest of your life. You'll get to a state of great health faster through a combination of a positive mindset and right action. It is critical that you first take control of your thoughts and feelings about your overall health and then follow this up with the right steps to improve your overall health. Before we go further, I want to acknowledge and congratulate you for taking action and acquiring this book. Take a second to give yourself a pat on the back for doing this to improve your health and life. You've already built some great momentum. You're well on your way to building some wonderful new habits for yourself. Feel and visualize that virtual *high five* from me. You got this!

Let's keep this momentum going for the long haul. Start thinking of yourself as a healthy person. Start to feel what it would be like to be healthy all of the time and, if necessary, to be free of prescription drugs. Feel what it would be like to be able to do any sport, even as you age into the retirement years. Start to picture yourself as looking and feeling great when you're 40, 50, 60, 70, 80, 90 and 100 plus! Imagine people telling you that you look so good and asking for your secret. Affirm that you are healthy and happy. Believe that you are going to have fantastic results from following the recommendations laid out in these pages. Celebrate your success now! Be excited and feel good about your future!

One of my all-time favorite personal development authors is Dr. Wayne Dyer. Wayne was a special man and I had the good fortune of meeting him in person. When I was working in the corporate world, I lived in the Washington, D.C. area. I once had a business trip to Richmond, Virginia, where I had to spend the night. I have some good friends in Richmond and planned a dinner gathering with them. I remember sitting in the lobby of the hotel that first day reading the paper. I looked up for a moment, and in walks Wayne Dyer with his assistant. I immediately jumped out of my chair and walked up to the front desk area to introduce myself to him. I told him that I was a big fan and I asked him what brought him to Richmond. He told me that he was giving a talk at the historic theatre downtown that same evening and invited me to come. I told him that I had dinner plans but would do my best to attend if I could.

Later that day I met up with my friends and we had a nice dinner. At the end of our dinner, I realized that I could make the talk but would probably miss the first 15 minutes of it. I hurried downtown and parked. I walked into this beautiful old theatre was greeted by a woman sitting at a desk who accepted tickets. I informed her that I met Wayne earlier in the day and he had invited me to come to his talk. I started to reach for my wallet when the woman got up and said, "Come with me." I followed her and she took me into the theater which was packed with people. While Wayne was on stage sharing his wisdom, she led me down the aisles to the only noticeable empty seat motioned for me to sit there. I thanked her and then sat down with gratitude as I contemplated what had just happened.

I thoroughly enjoyed his talk and left the theatre with a few extra kicks in my steps. There was something he said that night which really stood out for me. We've all heard the phrase; *I'll believe it when I see it.* Wayne shared how this phrase limits us from experiencing our full potential and the best way to get what you want is to shift your perspective to: *You'll see it when you believe it.* I've really come to understand in my life the truth of this statement. You won't believe you have great health after you see great health. It will never happen that way. You first have to believe that you have great health with all your heart, mind and soul. You have to think, feel and believe you have great health before it shows up in your life. You have to get a picture of yourself with great health in your mind and stick with before you see evidence of it. You'll then be led to take the necessary steps to take to make it happen, and eventually you'll experience long and lasting great health. It's the internal knowingness that will draw to you the results that you want. In fact, I would like to suggest that we change the affirmative thought to: *You'll see it when you know it!*

Before we move onto the actual steps for eliminating mouth sores, I want to discuss best practices for how to deal with them while you're still experiencing them. When you get these painful sores, you're willing to try anything. Well, believe me, I've tried just about every cure you can imagine. I've tried natural remedies, prescription drugs and over the counter products. None of these things were very effective at providing me with immediate relief. I kept searching while holding onto the belief that there had to be something that was natural and effective at providing some fast relief.

I finally discovered Myrrh which is a resin extracted from a shrub called Commiphora, which is common in arid regions of Africa and Arabia. It's a liquid that is easily obtainable from an online retailer. Myrrh has been used throughout our ancient history as a perfume, incense and medicine. I don't know about you, but I like the idea of using an ancient medicine, something that has been used for hundreds or thousands of years. Myrrh works best at the beginning stages of a mouth sore. It is important for you to start to become more aware when you have any feelings of discomfort in your mouth. Allow me to emphasize; start paying attention every single day as to that state of affairs happening inside your mouth. If you start to feel any discomfort or pain, get to a bathroom mirror and, using a flashlight, thoroughly evaluate the area in question. Look all around the area for any signs of the beginning stages of a mouth sore.

If you are starting to get a mouth sore, the area of tissue in question is usually red and a little sore or painful and may or may not yet have a white center area. This is when you will want to take a cotton swab and dip it into the bottle of Myrrh and then thoroughly dab the area. You will feel some stinging but that will be your confirmation that, yes, this is definitely the beginning stage of a mouth sore. Dab the area for a few seconds and you should then see a lot of the redness and swelling start to dissipate. You'll want to keep doing this periodically throughout each day until the pain goes away and the sore starts to heal on its own. I recommend that you dab the area between meals, after meals and right before you go to sleep at night. If you catch the mouth sore at the beginning stage, it will help prevent it from increasing in size and spreading. It will also expedite the healing process.

If you already have a full-blown mouth sore before using the Myrrh, it's not quite as effective. This is because the sore has already reached its critical stage. It will, however, help with managing the pain and aid in the healing process. So, keep using it regardless. A few words of caution: make sure you give yourself a thorough examination. A dentist mirror can be helpful in some these instances. There have been times where I had discomfort in my mouth and when I checked my mouth, I couldn't find anything. I would fluff it off as perhaps being some food stuck in my teeth. After ignoring it for a while, the pain seemed to increase. When I went back and did a more thorough examination, I would discover a full-blown mouth sore in a hard-to-see area. Train yourself to become more sensitive to any discomfort inside your mouth. Be proactive and immediately and thoroughly evaluate the area. Keep a good flashlight near your bathroom.

Whenever I bite my cheeks by mistake, I always dab some Myrrh on there to reduce the swelling, aid in the healing process and as a preventative measure for mouth sores. In fact, when I experience any trauma to my mouth, I dab some Myrrh on the affected area right away. Be aware that it does have a bitter taste. The Myrrh will likely cause your mouth to salivate a bit and it's good to swish this mixture around in your mouth before spitting it out as a preventative measure.

To see what kind of Myrrh I use and recommend, check out my website at cankersorecure.com. I've created this resource for you as a one-stop shop resource for all the products that I've used to help me manage and eliminate mouth sores.

So, now we're about to embark on the next journey of our time together where we start taking the steps to achieve mouth sore-free, great health. Before we go any further, I want to emphasize that this is not an overnight fix. Yes, some of the things that you'll be doing may give you some immediate relief from experiencing them. However, in order to achieve a significant reduction or the complete elimination of them, you have to be patient and follow all of the steps as laid out in this protocol. I recommend that you give this approach at least six months to experience the best results. The longer the better.

Do your best to follow this protocol as accurately as you can, but remember that our bodies are different, so you may find that doing more of X instead of Y may be more effective for you. That being said, I am confident that if you closely follow the process as outlined in the forthcoming chapters, you'll have a dramatic reduction of mouth sores with the lovely byproduct of being much healthier than you are today. And, as a wonderful side benefit, you may find that any other ongoing health issue you've been having will likely fall by the wayside. You'll be more energetic, happier and healthier.

You get to choose the level of health you want to have. You may not be willing to sacrifice some of the food and drink that I recommend that you eliminate, even if it's during a trial period. As your mentor, I want you to step up to the plate and aim for the home run. I'm giving you the big, fat, juicy pitches with this game plan. I'm asking you to give it a chance and swing for the fence.

Why settle for less? Don't you deserve the best health? Your body is your temple and will appreciate you treating it as such. And heck, if you end up with a triple rather than a home run, is that so bad?

Start creating a vision of yourself living a long and healthy life and rarely ever getting any sickness or disease. You can do this! I believe in you. Do you believe in you?

CHAPTER 4

<u>Step One:</u> Eliminate Certain Foods

"Knowing what must be done does away with fear"
- Rosa Parks

As we move into our game plan to silence these nasty mouth sores, let's go after the low hanging fruit first. Step One will be to temporarily eliminate eating foods that are known to cause an outbreak of mouth sores. Let me clarify what I mean when I use the word "temporarily." At some point you will be able to reintroduce some of these foods back into your diet to see whether they still cause issues for you. Some of these foods will ultimately be very good for you to eat. You may choose to reintroduce a certain food at a later date and may find that you can continue consuming it without any problem. If the food you have reintroduced causes an outbreak, you'll then know to avoid it and perhaps attempt to reintroduce it into your diet at a later time. All this means is that your body needs more time to heal. Or, if you are really brave, you may continue to live with a sore now and then just so you can still eat the item that is still causing an issue. You have to decide your level of tolerance. I believe if you stick with this plan for the long term, you will be able to reintroduce many of the healthy foods that are known triggers of mouth sores.

You already know my story. I'm not interested in ever having another mouth sore if there is anything that I can do about it. I didn't want them in the past and I continue to be willing to whatever it takes to be free of them. This determination has led me to sacrificing a few things in my diet that I thought I would never ever sacrifice. I thought about easing you into this first one, but why wait? I think you can handle it. You'll ultimately decide if you want to eliminate it or not. This may not be a big deal for you but for many people will be tough thing to let go.

Okay, enough suspense already. If you haven't guessed it already, I'm talking about eliminating drinking alcohol of every kind. I know, I can hear you screaming right now: "no way! I'm not giving this up!" I get it, however, I want you to hear me out. Of all the things that can cause mouth sores, I believe alcohol to be the biggest direct and indirect cause of them all. Alcohol is an immune system suppressant. I don't believe that any amount of alcohol is good for you. You hear a lot about drinking in moderation. I don't think so. I believe even one or two drinks per week is not healthy for you. There is a lot of supportive documentation to back me up. This is especially true if you have any kind of immune deficiency disorder. And, if you're reading this book, there is a good chance you are one of these people.

Let me share a story with you. I had been cranking along following my plan as outlined in this book. I had proudly gone about six months without having an alcoholic drink of any kind and I hadn't experienced a mouth sore for that same amount of time. I was feeling great. Before I go further, I don't want you to think I was an alcoholic or I drank all of the time because that was never the case with me (with the exception of my college years.) I was a social drinker and might have a glass of wine or two on the weekends. I had always equated drinking with being social. I never really liked how I felt the next day after a couple of drinks, but it was important for me to have a drink or two when socializing. Perhaps you can relate to this. It's a big, limiting belief for many people.

Society has done a great job of nudging us into bad habits. Alcohol is a multi-billion dollar industry. We tend to emulate society. Look at all of those ads and movies with the beautiful people dressed so eloquently with a drink in their hand. They're usually in a mansion smiling and laughing while attending an over-the-top cocktail party. I'm sure that you get the picture here and how we equate consuming alcohol with being beautiful, happy and rich. Drinking alcohol is made to be the thing to do if you want to be cool like these people. I bought into this mindset hook, line and sinker. So, you can imagine how hard it was for me to let go of this image of myself.

Getting back to the story, it had been six months since I had a drink or a mouth sore. We were attending our second wedding out of state in as many months. At the first wedding, as tempting as it was, I did not have one drink. I was really proud of myself. However, after six months without an alcoholic drink, either I got a little weaker at the knees or I got a bit cocky (or both.) I started having second thoughts and was pondering having a drink again to test the waters. My wife, Nancy, was rarely drinking at this point because she didn't like the effects it had on her and partly to support me. She is a sweetie! This second wedding was in Charlottesville, North Carolina and we had made a four-day mini-vacation out of it. A bit of my social anxiety started to creep back into my brain.

Both Nancy and I knew that this was going to be a really nice wedding held at the posh country club in Charlottesville, North Carolina. My favorite drink has always been a gin and tonic, Tanqueray[3] and tonic to be exact. I would always tell people that gin is good for you. Gin comes from juniper and juniper has medicinal properties. Also, tonic water has quinine in it which has been used to treat infections like malaria. I would tell people that, because of these two ingredients, gin and tonics are healthy for you. I did a great job of rationalizing how drinking a gin and tonic was harmless.

It was the day before the wedding, we were having lunch and I reminded my wife about gin being so good for people. We both started researching gin on our cellphones and guess what? We found article after article about how good gin is for you. I wonder who sponsored these articles. We then proceeded to get ourselves all jazzed up about having a drink at the wedding which was coming up on the next day. I thought this would be a good test for me. If I didn't get a mouth sore soon after consuming a gin and tonic, I might be able to drink again or at least have a Tanqueray and tonic on occasion. Well, we didn't even make it to the wedding before we both had our first alcoholic drink in a long time. That night, we were in the hotel lobby and they had this drink special with gin and some other liqueur and it sounded pretty good. We both got one and we really enjoyed them. We were practicing for the wedding the next day. That was the plan until I woke the next day with a mouth sore. I kid you not. I couldn't believe it. I had nothing to eat that I had been avoiding so I knew it was related to the alcohol.

---

[3] Tanqueray Gin, manufactured by Diageo Plc

I was so bummed to say the least. So, we attended this beautiful wedding and I obviously did not have a drink. In fact, I have not had a drink since that day and I'm now completely over the social anxiety thing. Pain and suffering have a way of doing this to you.

This entire experience was a huge blessing for me. Here's why: I don't want to get mouth sores and I am healthier because I do not consume alcohol. I know how alcohol affects the body. I believe I'm going to live longer and be happier because of this decision. I feel really good about it. I feel like I finally conquered it. If I'm at an event and someone asks me if I would like a drink, I proudly and confidently tell them, "no thank you, I don't drink." Instead, I'll get a sparkling water with lime on ice and I'm good to go. In a funny and ironic way, I used to be envious of people who didn't drink even though I felt strongly about drinking socially. Now I get to be that person I was so envious of in the past. Pretty cool how life works sometimes. The best part of all this is that I can still be sociable and then I always feel fantastic the next day. No more hangovers for me. This is a beautiful win-win result.

If I haven't convinced you yet to give up alcohol at least temporarily while you're resetting your body, let me give you a little bit of science. We'll talk about the importance of a healthy diet in Chapter 6. One of the most important contributors to our overall health and what we eat is the gut microbiome. The gut microbiome consists of trillions of microorganisms made up of bacteria, viruses and fungi. These microorganisms are actually foreign to us. That's right, they are like little tiny aliens that live in our body that play a critical role in regulating the homeostasis of our body. The food we eat plays a significant role in diversity of the microbiome which then, in turn, plays a key role in regulating our immune system.

When we drink alcohol, the first place it goes is into our gastro-intestinal (GI) tract. Our GI tract consists of the mouth, esophagus, stomach and intestines. When it reaches our stomach, it affects the quality and numbers of microorganisms in our gut microbiome. If you think you get a little tipsy and incoherent when drinking alcohol, what do you think it is doing to these tiny organisms. We have a few pounds of these little aliens. Do you think it's possible that many of them get altered and possibly knocked out for good? It turns out that these microorganisms play a critical role in the quality of our immune system too. A recent study[4] demonstrated that alcohol can disrupt the communication between these organisms and parts of our immune system. Keep in mind that everything is connected within the GI tract. Therefore, if you're having a problem in one area of the GI tract, there's a strong likelihood that it is adversely affecting the other areas of the GI tract.

If you recall, when I had the allergic reaction to the sulfa-based antibiotic, my entire GI tract was affected. I had canker sores in my mouth and I also had them around my anus. I can't imagine what was going on with those microorganisms in my gut. I see now how the GI tract is so intertwined. This is a good time for me to tell you about another related health issue I was experiencing along with the mouth sores: I found that sometimes when I was dealing with mouth sores, I had pain and bleeding during bowel movements. Fun, eh? It turns out that I had an anal fissure which is like a small tear in your anal canal. This is different than the canker-like sores

---

[4] **ncbi.nlm.nih.gov; reference article PMC4590612**

I got when I had the allergic reaction to the antibiotic. It can be a little scary with the pain and the blood, however, like mouth sores, it is not considered by the medical profession to be a serious health issue. Regardless, it sure felt serious to me when I was in the midst of it all. Recurrent bouts of soreness and bleeding were pretty darn frustrating to me. The annal fissure problem eventually cleared up from my using some home-made essential oil suppositories before bed and following everything as outlined in this book.

I started to see a correlation in the timing of the mouth sores and symptoms from the anal fissure. It was beyond coincidental. I realized that something was going on with my immune system within the GI tract. This led me to do some research and try to figure how to strengthen my immune system. To sum up things, we need to be proactive and avoid things that can harm the immune system and GI tract at the same time we're consuming things to strengthen it. This will be a powerful one-two punch.

(Please note that I will make bold and underline the things to remove from your diet so you can easily find them as a reference. You will also find a list of these items as the end of this chapter.)

So, let me suggest that you remove **<u>all forms of alcohol</u>** from your diet for at least six months. I want to encourage you to give it a shot. Okay, forget that. Let's replace the word "shot" with the word "try." No shots allowed here! I want to encourage you to give a try and see how you feel. Trust me, your microbiome will love you for it. This one move alone can significantly reduce many of your health issues. That wouldn't be so bad, would it? Now that we got the toughest item out of the way, it's all downhill from here.

The next thing to eliminate from your diet is all **vinegar products**. You'll discover that many of the products you'll be eliminating are very acidic in nature. Mouth sores thrive in an acidic environment. Vinegar is one of the most acidic foods out there. You probably remember the story of how I got a mouth sore within 30 minutes of having a salad with red wine vinegar for the salad dressing. I now know that, at that time, my sensitivity level was high. I also know that our bodies are different. However, vinegar is a known cause of mouth sores. Remove all vinegar products from your diet including apple cider vinegar which is presented to us as a health product.

This next item was an easy one for me to eliminate from my diet. I'm not a fan of **spicy foods consisting of pepper spices**. I don't digest them well. According to a number of studies, over

half the population likes spicy foods. One popular hot sauce contains pepper and vinegar. Now, assuming you are prone to having mouth sores, if you ever want to create one for some reason, this might be a really good product to swish around in your mouth for a few minutes. I'm guessing that you will not be volunteering for that experiment. Pepper spices are highly acidic, and they likely will exacerbate a mouth sore if there is even the slightest sign of one in your mouth. Remember my burrito story? I want to clarify here that peppers can be good for your overall health. And perhaps eating fresh cut peppers is okay. However, for people suffering from chronic mouth sores, I recommend that pepper spices be temporarily removed from the diet.

One spicy food that I love is ginger. Ginger is very alkaline and has many health benefits and is not known to cause mouth sores,

Ginger helps relieve inflammation so it might actually help prevent mouth sores. It is known to help prevent stomach ulcers, and a canker sore is a type of ulcer. We'll talk a lot more about diet in Chapter 6. I recommend you add ginger to your diet as much as possible. Ginger also relieves nausea and sea sickness. Whenever I go on a cruise, I always take a bottle of ginger capsules with me. Ginger has been proven to be as effective as Dramamine[5] for preventing sea sickness. Many years ago, I was on a cruise with Nancy. This particular ship was smaller than the typical ocean liner and it donned sails. During the trip, we encountered some rough waters and a number of people started getting nauseous and sick. I, however, had come prepared and started taking ginger root immediately. I never once felt nauseous. I was handing it out to my friends like candy. I chuckle because, one night, I had a knock on my cabin door from a complete stranger who had heard about this "magical herb" and then made the effort to track me down. I happily gave him a bunch of capsules to reward him for his efforts.

If you are a chronic sufferer of mouth sores, you will want to **limit your intake of citrus fruits, especially lemons, limes, oranges and grapefruit**. These citrus fruits do have an alkalizing effect once they are digested and metabolized into your body. In that regard, they are very good for you as they help to raise the pH of your body. However, outside of your body, these citrus fruits are acidic in nature. Same goes for when you first place them into your mouth. If your immune system is down or if there is even the

---

[5] **Dramamine is a registered trademark of Prestige Consumer Healthcare and is a drug used for motion sickness, nausea and dizziness**

slightest mouth sore brewing in there, eating a lot of citrus fruit might cause problems.

I thought I could beat the system and drink lemon water every day. I would squeeze half of a lemon into a 24-ounce Ball jar and drink it with a straw so it would minimize it touching my mouth tissue. I knew lemon is one of the most alkalizing foods you can eat when it is processed inside your body. I thought if I could raise the pH in my body, I would not get mouth sores as often. Well, check this little experiment off your to do list because I was still getting mouth sores every month. I came to the conclusion that the lemon water inside my mouth was exacerbating any sores that were percolating. Needless to say, I stopped drinking lemon water for the time being.

Other fruits that have been known to cause mouth sores are **pineapple and strawberries**. For me personally, strawberries never seemed to cause a problem, but I still decided to limit my intake of them. On the other hand, pineapple did cause a problem for me. I found a correlation between eating pineapple and getting a mouth sore to two. I want to reiterate that our bodies are different and that you'll need to figure which foods are aggravating your body system and causing problems for you. Or, you can take the safe way by temporarily eliminating all of the foods that are known causes of mouths sores.

Tomato is widely known as a vegetable but technically is a fruit. I don't care to get into the politics of what it is, but I do recommend that you temporarily **eliminate tomato and tomato sauce from your diet**, at least for six months. I'm Irish and English by my ancestry but I must have some Italian in me because two of favorite foods in the world have always been pizza and spaghetti. My mother used to make the best spaghetti and meatballs in the world. She once gave me her recipe, but I could never make it as good as she could. So, if you're bummed about not being able to eat these two foods for a while, believe me, I can relate. Know that if you follow the protocol in this book, you will heal, and you will be able to eat these foods again. I can attest to this fact.

I've shared the story of how I tried to cheat my way back to having and drink or two with the gin and tonic. That did not turn out well for me. Well, I have another story for you. I was enjoying not having to deal with mouth sores for a long time but that Italian nature in me kept prodding me. I really missed eating traditional pizza and spaghetti. After being on my healing protocol for a few months, my wife mentioned that she was going to make some bean soup and asked me if it would be okay to throw in some tomato sauce. I thought it would likely be harmless and I told her to go ahead and do it. It seemed like a good time to try and reintroduce tomatoes as I know they are so good for us. She asked me if I was sure about it. I gave her the affirmative. Well, she made a huge pot of this Italian bean soup and we ended up eating it 3 days in a row.

You're probably surmising what happened next. Yep, right after the third day I got a mouth sore. Because my body was healing and I had been following this protocol for a few months, I only got one sore and it cleared up twice as fast. However, it was another sign for me to stay away from tomato of any kind for a little while longer. I'm guessing that if I had eaten the soup only one night, I might have been okay. It was eating tomato for three nights in a row that probably did it. Once again, it is important to at least temporarily stop eating foods that are potential causes of mouth sores. You will be able to reintroduce them again in the future to see if they cause you problems. I recommend that you go at least six months without eating these foods. I know you can do this because you know that pain and discomfort involved with having multiple mouth sores. Why not beat these buggers once and for all or, at the very least, make it a rare occurrence? I eat tomatoes all the time now and I never get a mouth sore.

Other foods that have been suspect causes of mouth sores are **<u>cinnamon, wheat/gluten, chocolate and sugary products like soda</u>**. I have to admit, being a chocolate love, I never gave it up because it never seemed to cause a problem for me. If you are like me, then perhaps you could continue to eat chocolate on occasion to see if it causes a problem. However, be aware, if you do get a mouth sore right after consuming some chocolate, you might be one of the "unlucky" ones and have to give it up for six months to a year. As part of the transformation of my diet over time, I now only eat chocolate made with natural sweeteners like stevia. Stevia is a natural herb. I don't eat any artificial or refined sugars. We'll talk more about sugar later in the book.

Below you will see two lists of foods to avoid. The first list is the "No Go" list. I recommend that you eliminate these foods from your diet for at least six months as you reset your body. Some of these foods are good for you such as lemon, oranges and the other fruits listed there. Yet, when you are dealing with chronic mouth sores, you want to avoid these healthy foods for a while as they are acidic in nature while inside the mouth. The second list is the

"Low Go" list, meaning that I recommend that you don't eat any of these foods or very little of them for the next six months. It's up to you as to how far you want to take this plan.

"No Go" List

Pineapple
Orange
Lemon
Lime
Grapefruit
Strawberry
Tomato
Tomato Sauce
Spicy Foods
Pepper spices
Soda
Toothpaste with SLS (Sodium Lauryl Sulfate)

"Low Go" List

Peanut Butter
Acidic Foods
Dairy Products
Wheat/Gluten Products
Coffee
Cinnamon
Processed Foods
Chocolate

CHAPTER 5

<u>Step Two:</u> Drink Healthy Water

"Water is the only drink for a wise man"
- Henry David Thoreau

You're probably wondering why I'm devoting an entire chapter to water. You may be thinking that water is water and all water is good for us. Well, not exactly. Our bodies are comprised mostly of water. In fact, more than 50% of our bodyweight is comprised of water with the average being between 50 and 65%. Water plays a many different roles in the proper functioning of our bodies, all of which are critical to our overall health. Here is a list of the some of the things water does for us:

- It facilitates the digestion of food and conversion of food into energy

- It's used by cells to transfer certain chemicals between one and another

- It helps our body regulate a proper body temperature via perspiration

- It plays a key role in our waste removal system

- It's a lubricant for our tissue and joints

If water plays such critical role in our overall health and our bodies are comprised mostly of it, it makes sense to drink a lot of it. This will ensure that our body is functioning at peak potential. I urge you to look at water as the most important substance you can ingest. To accomplish this, start paying close attention to the amount of water you drink each and every day.

The quality of the water you drink is just as important as the amount of water you drink. I do not recommend drinking tap water. Our local municipality tells us it's safe and harmless to drink and that's it been tested for impurities. I'm not buying it. For one, they add a bunch of chemicals to it such as chlorine and fluoride. They started adding fluoride to our water back in the 1940's to help prevent tooth decay. Fluoride has been found to be a neurotoxin. It can have an adverse effect on the thyroid and pineal gland. Many countries have banned water fluoridation. That should tell you something. Chlorine is a chemical that is typically used as a cleaning agent because it prevents bacteria growth in water. If enough chlorine gets in your gut, chemical reactions can occur producing hydrochloric acid which is a poisonous substance to humans.

When your local water plant "purifies" the water, they test it right there on location and they give you the test results that show very little contaminants. They don't talk about things like fluoride and chlorine because those chemicals are considered safe by them. This "purified" drinking water then has to pass from the water plant through miles of rusty old pipes to and throughout your house. A lot of our country's water infrastructure is old. There is still a lot of lead piping in the ground. Lead has been found in our water supply and it is toxic to our body. Who knows what contaminates are polluting the water on its way to your house. Pesticides have also been known to seep into the water lines. Nobody tests the water once it reaches your house. I bet if it was tested, you would get much different results than what they get at the plant. Other toxins that have been found in our country's water supply have been mercury, dioxins, herbicides, arsenic and perchlorate.

I could go on and on about the dangers of drinking tap water. I'll stop here. Don't take a chance on your health with one of the most important ingredients you can put in your body. It doesn't cost that much to drink purified or good natural spring water Look at it as a really good investment in your overall health.

I've been a healthy water advocate for a long time. We raised our kids mostly in Colorado. Living in Colorado meant having access to some of the best natural spring water in the country.

The water that emanates from The Rocky Mountains has been filtered naturally through layers of ground and minerals for thousands of years. It's some of the crispest, freshest water I've ever had.

Knowing how important it is to drink, good, healthy water, I wondered how my family would react if I purchased a water cooler and some spring water delivered to my house. We figured it would make a positive difference, so we went ahead and purchased one of the top-end water coolers with the instant hot water feature and safety valve. We knew if the kids drank more water, there would likely be less doctor visits. As thoughtful parents, we wanted our three children to be as healthy as possible. This theory seemed to play out very well because our kids started drinking a lot more water. We did start to notice a drop off in sickness and doctors' visits. Also, our kids came to appreciate water and they hardly drank anything else. Same for my wife and me.

Fast forward a few years (okay, 18 years) to when we became empty nesters. Our adult children all moved to California to pursue their dreams and my wife and I decided to give Texas a try. We have some family in the state and wanted a break from shoveling snow. Right after we moved to Texas, one of the first things I did was to look for a good source of natural spring water. I was relieved to find that there was something called Texas spring water and I could have it delivered to my house. I bought a brand new, fancy water cooler and put it right beside the refrigerator. It was stainless steel and it even had oxidation feature to purify the water lines. It looked pretty sweet. I started getting the water delivered and it tasted pretty good as far as I could tell. Not as good as the Colorado water but it tasted fine.

We have a swimming pool at our house and so I had purchased a pH test kit for the pool so I could monitor the pH levels of the pool water. After having this spring water delivered for a couple of months, I noticed the pH kit sitting inside a cabinet collecting dust since we were using a pool service company. I got this spark of an idea to test the pH level of the spring water. I was certain that it would test above pH level of 7, which would mean it was alkaline water. I opened the kit and performed the test in anticipation of getting a great result. I was a little shocked to discover that this Texas spring water was highly acidic in nature. I was spending $30 per month to get acidic water delivered to my house. I picked up the phone and called the company and told them to cease delivery. I remember how strange it was that the customer service agent did not seem that surprised. I guess they knew this and figured most customers would never figure this out. This was the only spring water option in town. I did not want to pay for purified water delivery, which was another option. If I was going to be drinking purified water, I wanted to figure out how to do it on my own.

I spent a couple of weekends online looking and researching all available options for in-home water purification. There were many different kinds of options with a wide range of prices. Everything from whole-house filtration systems, bulky, under-the sink filtration systems, reverse osmosis systems, to over-the-counter electrolysis machines. Nothing seemed to be perfect. I was looking for an inexpensive and simple solution. I knew that there had to be something out there. I also wanted something that I would remove 99.99% of all contaminants and toxins. My ideal system would be able to alkalize the water.

The closest thing I could find to what I wanted was a water ionization appliance that alkalizes the water. They cost thousands of dollars and they don't do a fantastic job of filtering out all of the contaminants and toxins. Plus, you have to have this bulky machine sitting on your counter. My wife and I really didn't want to see a bulky appliance on the counter by our sink. I kept searching and I was about to give up when I just happened to come across an under-the-sink filtration system that not only removes all of the impurities but also alkalizes the water. And the best part is that it was very affordable. This system had already been successfully used in Mexico and was just being introduced into the United States.

I purchased it and it was fairly easy to set it up. We've been very happy with and I was so thrilled to find something so effective and inexpensive. (If you would like to learn what I'm using, please visit my website at cankersorecure.com. This site is a nice consolidation of all of the resources that I use.) If you do have spring water in your area, ask the providing company for the pH level of the water. They should be able to show you detailed test results of the pH and levels of impurities. To be alkaline, it needs to have a pH greater than 7. If you get spring water delivered to your house, you could get an inexpensive pH test kit and test it yourself to make sure it matches what they share with you.

Let's move on to how much water you should drink every day. It's worth noting that we lose a lot of water every day through urination, breathing, sweating and bowel movements. We do get some water from the food we eat but we need to make sure we are getting plenty of water to replace what we lose. This will ensure that our body system is firing on all cylinders. The name of the game is to be as healthy as possible.

Your body weight is an important factor when determining your water intake. There are many different recommendations out there for how much water to drink. One that I particularly like is from Dr. Sharon E. Griffin who holds a B.S., M.S., and Ph.D. in the areas of exercise science and physiology. She also holds a second M.S. degree in nutrition and is a certified health and fitness instructor. She knows her stuff. Her guideline is very simple and easy to remember, and it makes good common sense. Dr. Griffin states that, daily, you need to drink one-half ounce of water for every pound of body weight. If you weight 160 pounds, this would equate to 80 ounces of water or eight 10-ounce glasses per day. If you weight 140 pounds, this would mean you should drink seven 10-ounce glasses per day. This is an excellent guideline to follow.

I have a few tips I would like to share with you to help ensure you get a good amount of water per day. It is easy for us to get caught up in the minutiae of the day and forget to drink a lot of water. I've created a few habits to ensure that I drink plenty of water every day. First, as soon as I wake up in the morning and get out of bed, I walk to the kitchen and I fill up a large glass with 20 ounces of water. I then drink it over the next 15 minutes. Boom! I've already got 20 ounces of my total for the day. Another reason I do this is to rehydrate my body after 7-8 hours of sleep. We drink very little water at night while sleeping if any at all. I find that drinking this this glass of water first thing in the morning gets the body system fired up and it signals the digestive system to kick in gear to help eliminate the wastes that have been accumulating while we sleep. I believe drinking 16 to 20 ounces glass of water when you first wake up in the morning is one the best and easiest things you can do for your health.

The second thing I do is fill a glass with about 12 ounces of water right after I eat breakfast with the goal of drinking it and perhaps more before lunch. I'll either do this or make a cup of herbal tea. I usually wait an hour after eating my meals before drinking water or tea to allow the food in my stomach to digest properly. You do not want to dilute your digestive juices. There are a number of studies that demonstrate too much liquids during meals or immediately following meals can impede proper digestion. These first two habits put my total at roughly 36 ounces. I typically go for a run before lunch and usually end up drinking more water afterwards. If you exercise, be sure you are drinking a lot of water before, during and after to counter the loss of water through sweating.

The third healthy water habit that I practice is drinking 24 ounces of water after lunch and before dinner. We like to drink out of 24-ounce Ball mason jars. I like how they have indicators on them for different levels of ounces. Right after lunch I fill up one of these jars with water and take it to my office. I make sure that I drink this entire jar of water before dinner. Again, I usually don't start drinking it until about an hour after I eat. I have usually met my recommended water intake level for my body weight by dinnertime. I usually drink more than the recommended amount for my body weight as I am not counting extra cups of tea and smoothies. I drink very little water after dinner because I don't want to be up more than once per night to relieve myself. Get those water intake goals done by dinner so you can sleep soundly at night!

If you follow these three healthy water habits, you are setting a strong foundation for the amount of daily water you drink and you're more likely going to achieve your water intake goal. You will be drinking about 60 ounces of water every day without thinking too much about it. By doing these things, I've become very conscious of the amount of water that I drink on a daily basis. When you start to do this, you'll become more conscious as well. I'll drink to that! Pure, healthy water, of course.

One final note about water: as I was writing this book, I discovered the benefits of drinking distilled water. There is a lot of confusion out there as to whether or not distilled water is good for you. Many scientific experts state that distilled water is a neutral water based on the fact that the three atoms involved, H2O (one Hydrogen and two Oxygen atoms,) have an equal number of negative and positive charges. Thus, they cancel each other out creating a water structure that is neither negative nor positive but rather neutral. However, after digging deeper, I discovered through the work of Marina Jacobi[6] that the structure of distilled water changes after interacting with our body. In conjunction with the spinning of the molecular structure of every human being, the distilled water is transferred (recharged) into a negative charge as it comes into contact with the unnatural toxins in the body. This is because of two reasons: first, water has memory and can modify itself into a different platform of structure and, and second, the toxins have a higher negative charge over any other natural molecular substance in our body. The distilled water is a conductor, which means it will mimic the structure of the higher negative charge of the toxins by increasing its molecular spin rates, and then proceed to flush these toxins out of the body.

Store-bought distilled water in a plastic jug is fine to drink because, as previously shared, it will work to remove any toxins that have seeped into the water from the plastic container. The backers of drinking distilled water suggest starting out by drinking it one to three days at a time to allow your body the ability to gradually remove some toxins. I started out by drinking only distilled water as my liquid intake for three straight days. I sensed it was remov-

---

[6] **marinajacobi.com, 'The Harmonic Reactor' youtube.com channel, Season 2, Episode 17, Quantum Manifestation, Distilled Water Hz**

ing some toxins because I had some itchiness on my lower legs after a couple of days. I know toxins are always looking for ways to the exit the body and, when this happens, it's common for you to see signs of this on your skin. Since that initial three-day period, I've been drinking distilled water in the morning for my first large glass of water. I also like to repeat the three-day distilled water protocol at least once per month. Drinking purified, alkaline water and alternating with distilled water now is a powerful combination to add essential minerals and remove toxins.

CHAPTER 6

Step Three: A Diet for a Strong Immune System

"The first wealth is health."
- Ralph Waldo Emerson

Let's take a moment to assess where we are on this journey together for creating optimal health in our mouth and body. We've temporarily eliminated the foods that are the biggest culprits for causing mouth sores. You might have already noticed some relief if you're someone dealing with chronic sores. We then took steps to ensure that we are drinking only purified or good spring water. I realize that you may have not had the chance to do this yet. Please make it a priority. Keep on reading but do make a note to look into this as soon as possible. In order to get the best results from this program, you have to be willing to follow most if not all of these recommendations. They may seem like little things but know that the little things are the big things. Following all of the steps in this book will make a significant and positive impact in your health and life.

We've already discussed the importance of eating foods that are alkaline in nature and reducing foods that are acidic in nature. Studies show that mouth sores tend to thrive in an acidic environment. All of the foods we are temporarily eliminating (listed at the end of Chapter 4) are highly acidic while inside the mouth before they flow through the digestive tract to the stomach. This further proves that there is something behind this theory of acidic foods facilitating a breakout of mouth sores. I know from my own personal experience that certain acidic foods can trigger an outbreak of mouth sores. Acidic foods are more likely to weaken the immune system and most alkaline foods strengthen the immune system. This program is about becoming more aware of the foods that you're eating to ensure that our eating more alkaline foods and less acidic foods. See Figures 6.1 and 6.2 at the end of this chapter for separate lists of alkaline forming and acid forming foods.

There's a reason your parents wanted you to eat more vegetables when you were little: they knew vegetables were good for you. Most vegetables have a high level of alkalinity and are great for your immune system. You didn't think I was going to tell you that eating donuts is really good for your immune system, did you? If that were the case, I can assure you that they wouldn't taste like the donuts we know. They would probably be much less appetizing. The majority of people know if a certain food is good for them or not. We know that fresh food is much better for us than processed food. We know that vegetables and fruits are better for us than cookies and ice cream. However, as with any food you consume, there is more than meets the eye. There is another factor to consider in our diet that is just as important as eating more alkaline foods. Before we get into specific foods to eat, I would like to shed light on this mystery thing that may be wreaking havoc on your immune system.

While on this journey of eliminating mouth sores and improving my overall health, I discovered some incredible information

about the underlying cause of most health problems we face today;
health problems such as:

~ Mouth sores

~ Mononucleosis

~ Chronic Fatigue Syndrome

~ Adrenal fatigue

~ Lime disease

~ Fibromyalgia

~ Hormonal imbalances

~ Autoimmune disease

~ Depression

~ Thyroid problems

~ Chronic inflammation

~ Multiple Sclerosis

~ Neurological conditions

~ Hashimoto's disease

~ Acne

~ Eczema

~ Gut problems

~ Migraines

~ Psoriasis

You may discover that eating tomatoes or tomato sauce triggers a breakout of mouths sores for you but what is the reason that
this very healthy food would cause this to happen? If most people
can eat tomatoes and take in all the health benefits without any
adverse effects, why do you not experience the same? Wanting to

solve this mystery inspired me to keep digging until one day the answer came effortlessly to me.

Through her process of getting certified as a health coach, my wife discovered Anthony William, aka the Medical Medium[7]. When Anthony was four years old, God spoke to him through what he calls the Spirit of Compassion. He relays that initially he could see this Spirit but then, as he got older, he could only hear it. Imagine being four years old and having a conversation with God. When this first started happening, this Spirit told him to get up off his chair at the dinner table and walk over and stand by his grandmother. It then told him to place his hand over her chest and says these words, "Grandma, you have lung cancer." Anthony proceeded to do this and, needless to say, his entire family was quite shocked. His grandmother seemed perfectly healthy and they all wondered how he even knew about lung cancer at such a young age. The next week his grandmother went for a checkup and sure enough, she was diagnosed with lung cancer.

This was the beginning of Anthony's life-long journey to helping people heal from their medical problems. He can look at anybody and, without hesitation, tell them exactly what's going on in their body and what health issues they are dealing with. Anthony has written many best-selling books that talk about the most common health problems and how to heal them.

According to Anthony, the number one underlying cause of most health issues today is the Epstein-Barr virus (EPV.) EPV is a herpes related virus and the vast majority of people are carrying

---

[7] **medicalmedium.com**

the virus. It's one of nine human herpesviruses. EPV spreads mostly through saliva but it can also be passed from mother to baby during pregnancy. Experts may dispute this fact, but Anthony says a lot of his information about EPV is ahead of its time and science will someday prove him to be right. Anthony likes to reiterate that most health problems you face are not your fault. EPV is the main reason why.

I always wondered why I followed such a healthy lifestyle and yet I was dealing with chronic mouth sores. After reading Anthony's books, I was so relieved to finally understand why this was happening to me. I believe that those of us dealing with mouth sores are experiencing how EPV expresses itself in our bodies. There may be other issues at play when it comes to our health, however, I believe that EPV is the main underlying issue. This is because it weakens the immune system to create fertile ground for manifesting things like mouth sores and other health problems.

Now that we know that EPV is likely the main culprit for our health issues, what does Anthony suggest we do to heal ourselves? Well, it's all about the diet and eating the right healing foods. Anthony encourages us to primarily eat a plant-based diet with lots of healthy fruits and vegetables. Some fruits and vegetables have a greater healing effect over others. Anthony suggests that it's okay to eat some meat as long as it is grass-fed and it's okay to eat certain fish as long as it is wild-caught. Anthony explains that certain fruits and vegetables will have the most beneficial impact in your healing process. One such food is celery juice. Celery is technically an herb rather than a vegetable and, according to Anthony, it is one of the most powerful healing foods on the planet. It can kill viruses such as EPV and other harmful bacteria and fungi in our bodies. Anthony recommends that you drink 16 ounces of celery juice every morning on an empty stomach. I do this 30 minutes after I drink that first 24-ounce glass of water and I don't eat my breakfast until about an hour afterwards. I have a slow metabolism. Anthony recommends you don't eat breakfast until at least 30 minutes after drinking the celery juice.

My wife and I started drinking celery juice every day and within a month or two we began to notice some detox effects. We both experienced itchy breakouts on our skin for many weeks. It was annoying but I happy to know that is was the EPV dying off inside our bodies and the resulting toxins working their way out. We also both experienced cold and flu-like symptoms in the beginning. Anthony explains in his work that all of these symptoms can be part of the detox process. We continue to drink celery juice every morning and it has simply become a vital part of our regular diet.

As part of the Medical Medium protocol, you will want to avoid certain foods that feed EPV in your bodies. Some of these foods are gluten, dairy, eggs, corn, soy, pork, farmed fish, meat that is not grass-fed, canola oil and refined sugar. My wife and I chose to eliminate all of these foods from our diet and I am so glad we did. You have to decide your comfort level with it but I highly recommend that you research Anthony and explore some of his books. See how his information resonates with you. He has many recipes in his books and the foods are delicious! We do not feel like we are sacrificing anything by following his diet recommendations. In fact, we are healthier and more fit than any other point in our lives.

I never thought I would be saying that I no longer eat refined sugar, but you don't need it to indulge in sweets. There are plenty of natural sweeteners that do not spike the blood sugar, strengthen EPV and weaken the immune system. You'll learn more about them later in this chapter. After we were on this diet for about a year, I posed this question to my wife. I asked her what she would do if say, a few years ago, someone said to her that her husband would never drink alcohol again or eat any food containing refined sugar. She said she would have fallen down on the floor rolling around with laughter. I believe her as I never thought that would happen to me either. I am grateful for all my life experience which has led me with the knowledge and wisdom I have today.

I want to caution you before you start to go online and research Anthony William. You might find some "reliable" sources trashing his diet recommendations. I read one of his books without knowing this. However, as I was reading the book, one of the first thoughts I had was that this way of eating would be a huge threat to the pharmaceutical and dairy industries. What good is big Pharma if we don't need their expensive drugs? This thought was confirmed when my wife did a little digging on her own. She came to me to share what she found, and I immediately told her what I just stated to you. She got it. It's not uncommon for these industries to pay people (trolls) to target these perceived threats online and write articles and post comments with the sole purpose of creating doubt in peoples' minds. Again, I want to encourage you to get one or two of his books that resonate with you and start there. My thoughts were, *I'm certainly not going to harm myself by eating more healthy fruits and vegetables and less gluten, dairy and refined sugar.* This was just common sense to me.

Remember when we talked about the gut microbiome and how important it is to our overall health? To refresh your memory, the microbiome consists of trillions of bacteria, viruses and fungi. They play a critical role in regulating the homeostasis of our body and immune system. I had previously discussed how drinking alcohol can wreak havoc on the microbiome. Let's look at the other end of the spectrum and explore what we can do to improve our microbiome. There are two kinds of foods that target the microbiome in a good way. These are Prebiotic foods and Probiotic foods. Prebiotic foods feed the healthy gut bugs (bacteria, etc.) and starve the bad gut bugs. The healthy gut bugs want healthy foods and the unhealthy gut bugs want unhealthy foods. Seems logical. When you get a craving for something such as a cookie, you likely believe that this craving is coming from your conscious mind. You think it's *you* wanting a cookie. However, science has demonstrated that it's the gut bugs in your microbiome that are signaling your brain to feed them what they want. If the bad bugs are in control, they want sugars and starches. If the good bugs are in control, they want healthy vegetables. I never thought I would crave a salad but after eating a primarily plant-based diet for six months, my mouth would start to water when I eyed a good salad. My wife and I eat a salad almost every day for lunch. We add in ingredients like cucumber, carrots, zucchini, yellow squash, apple, pistachios, nuts, chopped dates, and onions. We toss the salad and ingredients with a high-quality olive oil as the dressing with a pinch of sea salt. It's so good and fulfilling! When you get to the point when you crave a salad like this, you'll know that you are on the right track with your diet.

Here are some of the top healing fruits and vegetables:

Wild blueberries

Apples

Bananas

Figs

Raspberries

Pomegranates

Grapes

Papaya

Potatoes

Sweet Potatoes

Cucumber

Artichokes

Asparagus

Leafy Greens

Spinach

Onions

Cruciferous vegetables

Celery

Some great natural sugar substitutes that don't spike your blood sugar:

Coconut sugar

Raw honey

Maple syrup

Dates

I recommend that you add as much of these foods as possible to your diet. You'll be killing off EPV and increasing the number of good gut bugs in your microbiome.

Make sure that you're buying as much organic food as possible. You do not want to be eating foods containing pesticides as pesticides are poisons. Also, avoid GMO (genetically modified organism) food at all costs. Despite what you might read or hear in the media, GMO foods are not good for you. There are many studies now showing that GMO foods do damage to our bodies and increase the likelihood of disease. This stems from testing on animals which resulted in auto immune diseases, cancer, infertility, gastrointestinal disorders and organ failure. Also, be sure to stay away from artificial sweeteners in any food as they too can wreak havoc on your immune system. Many years ago, I came down with a strange autoimmune illness after drinking a sport powered drink for a month that had an artificial sugar in it. I wasn't aware it contained an artificial sugar because the artificial sugar was sucralose. I was thinking this ingredient was sucrose, which is regular sugar. They disguised the real sugar with a similar name. Sucralose has been shown to cause problems in your digestive system including the microbiome. It kills off the good bacteria and if there's any bad bacteria in there, it feeds them and helps them to proliferate. My particular illness lasted about a month and I had Mononucleosis-like symptoms. There are many stories of people getting ill after consuming artificial sugars for an extended period of time. Stay away from them. Finally, reduce your intake of processed foods as much as possible. They deprive your body of proper nutrients and are typically made with chemicals, artificial sweeteners and hydrogenated oils. If you buy any processed food, make sure to buy organic and be sure to read the ingredient labels.

Herbal teas have amazing medicinal benefits. People have been using the healing power of plants for thousands of years. Herbs are loaded with vitamins and vital nutrients. There are many herbal teas which aid our digestive system. As part of healing my gut, I researched them in detail and then created a 30-day tea protocol which I felt did an amazing job with helping to heal my gut. I used the following teas and ingredients:

Organic Fennel Tea - Fennel is well-known for its ability to soothe the gut and ease bloating and gassiness. It is a great aid for digestion as it helps to smooth the muscles of the gastrointestinal system.

Organic Licorice Root Tea - This is another great tea for supporting our digestive health. It is known for speeding up the repair of the stomach lining. It has anti-inflammatory and immune boosting properties.

Organic Marshmallow Root Powder - You might be wondering if I am referring to the common candy. Actually, the original marshmallow candy was made from the marshmallow plant roots. Unfortunately, the candy that we know of today no longer contains any marshmallow root and, instead, is made from sugar, egg whites and gelatin. Marshmallow root powder is high in anti-inflammatory properties and it moistens, soothes and supports the digestive tract. It has been used to treat stomach ulcers and has many other benefits such as providing pain relief, speeding up wound healing, reducing coughs and colds, and improving overall skin health.

<u>30-day Tea Healing Protocol</u> - This program is only recommended when you are not experiencing any mouth sores. Drinking hot liquids can irritate an active sore. I recommend purchasing only high-quality, organic teas and enough of each tea to last for 30 days. See my website (cankersorecure.com) for the type of teas I recommend. You can buy organic marshmallow root powder at various retailers online and one bag should be plenty enough for 30 days. With every cup of tea, include one or two scoops of the marshmallow root powder. Have the fennel tea in the morning between lunch and breakfast, alternate the teas between lunch and dinner and the licorice tea an hour after dinner as it will satisfy the sweet tooth urges. If three cups of tea per day are too much for you, try to drink a minimum of two cups of tea during the 30-day period. Also, if you are concerned about multiple trips to the bathroom at night, when preparing the last cup of tea, fill the cup with hot water to about 3/4ths its normal level.

Be very mindful of this protocol and try not to miss a scheduled cup of tea. Make reminders for yourself if necessary. You may find as I did that, after doing this for a few days, you'll truly start to enjoy drinking these teas and appreciate the value of their soothing, medicinal properties. Within a week of being on this protocol, I didn't have to worry about reminding myself because I looked forward to it so much.

At the end of the 30-day period, assess how you feel and, if necessary, continue the protocol for another two to four weeks. I was amazed at how great my stomach felt after one month. This protocol relieved the bloating and gas I was experiencing along with the slight feeling of discomfort that I had at the top area of my stomach for many years. This is something you can always go back and repeat, if necessary, in the years ahead. It's a wonderful healing modality and it should make a significant impact with reducing or eliminating your occurrence of mouth sores.

Certain supplements will help with preventing mouth sores and improving overall health. For example, people who suffer chronic sores are typically low in Folic Acid (B9) and B12. These two vitamins are important in red blood cell production. Below is a list of vitamins I recommend placed into two categories: Must Haves and Should Haves. I realize that purchasing supplements can be expensive so you will want to prioritize based on your personal budget. To see the products that I take and recommend, visit my website at cankersorecure.com.

MUST HAVES

Methyl Folate - Helps prevent mouth sores and improve immune system.

Methyl B12 - Also helps prevent recurrent mouth sores.

Zinc - Boosts immune system. Zinc deficiency can cause recurrent mouth sores.

Probiotics - Helps with the gut microbiome and digestive health.

Multivitamin - Helps to ensure you are getting proper vitamins for overall health.

SHOULD HAVES

Vitamin E - Great antioxidant that reduces free radical damage.

Flax, Fish or Krill Oil - Helps to reduce inflammation and improve skin.

Vitamin C - Helps improve immune system and repair body tissue.

L-Lysine - Helps boost immune system and prevent cold and mouth sores.

<u>Alkaline Forming Foods</u>

Alfalfa Grass
Almonds
Almond Milk
Aloe Juice
Amaranth
Apples
Apricots
Artichokes
Asparagus
Avocados
Baking Soda
Bananas
Barley Grass
Beet Greens
Beets
Bell Peppers
Blackberries
Blueberries
Broccoli
Brussel Sprouts
Buckwheat
Cabbage
Cantaloupe
Carrots
Cauliflower
Cayenne Pepper
Celery
Chard Greens
Cherries
Chestnuts
Chia Seeds
Chicory
Chives
Cilantro

Cinnamon
Coconut (fresh)
Coconut Water
Collard Greens
Comfrey
Cooked Broccoli
Cooked Spinach
Cucumbers
Cumin Seeds
Currants
Curry
Dandelion Greens
Dates
Dill
Distilled Water
Dulce
Edible Flowers
Eggplant
Endive
Fennel Seeds
Figs
Flax Seed Oil
Flax Seeds
Ginger Root
Grapefruit
Grapes
Green Beans
Green Cabbage
Green Tea
Guava
Hemp Seeds
Herbal Tea
Herbs
Honey

Honeydew
Horseradish
Jicama
Kale
Kiwi
Kohlrabi
Leeks
Lemons
Lentils
Lettuce
Limes
Mangoes
Melons
Millet
Mushrooms
Mustard Greens
Nectarines
Nigella Seeds
Okra
Olive Oil
Olives
Onions
Oranges
Papayas
Parsley
Parsnips
Pears
Peas
Peaches
Peppers
Pineapple
Poppy Seeds
Potatoes
Pumpkin

Pumpkin Seeds   Sesame Seeds   Tangerines
Primrose Oil   Sorrel   Taro Root
Quinoa   Spinach   Tomatoes
Radish   Spirulina   Turnips
Raisins   Sprouts   Water Chestnuts
Red Cabbage   Squashes   Watercress
Rhubarb   Stevia   Wheat Grass
Rutabaga   Strawberries   White Radish
Rosehips   Sunflower Oil   Wild Greens
Sea Salt   Sunflower Seeds Wild Rice
Seaweed   Sweet Potatoes Yams
Sesame   Tamari   Zucchini

Figure 6.1
Include as much of these foods as possible in your diet.

Acid Forming Foods

Agave
Artificial Sugars
Barley
Beef
Beer
Beet Sugar
Black Beans
Black Tea
Brazil nuts
Breads
Brown Rice
Butter
Buttermilk
Candy
Canned Foods
Canned Fruit
Canola Oil
Cakes
Carbonated Drinks
Carob
Cashews
Cereals
Cheeses
Chicken
Chickpeas
Chocolate
Clams
Cocoa
Coconut (dried)
Coconut Oil
Coffee
Cooked Beans
Cooked Tomatoes
Cooked Vegetable
Cookies

Corn
Corn Oil
Corn Starch
Corn Syrup
Crab
Cranberries
Cream
Dairy
Duck
Fish
Fried Foods
Fructose
Garbanzos
Goat Cheese
Goat Milk
Hazelnut
Honey
Ice Cream
Jams
Ketchup
Kidney Beans
Margarine
Molasses
Lamb
Lima Beans
Liquor
Liver
Lobsters
Kidney Beans
Macadamias
Mayonnaise
Milk
Molasses
Mustard
Navy Beans

Oat Milk
Oats
Oysters
Pasta
Pastries
Peanuts
Pecans
Pickles
Pinto Beans
Pistachios
Plums
Popcorn
Pork
Processed Foods
Processed Juices
Prunes
Rabbit
Rice Cakes
Rice Milk
Scallops
Salmon
Salted Butter
Shellfish
Soda
Soybeans
Soy Flour
Soy Milk
Soy Sauce
Spelt
Sprouted Wheat
Bread
Sugar
Sweetened Fruit
Juice
Table Salt

Tamari	Walnuts	Microwaved Foods
Tapioca	Watermelon	
Tomato Sauce	Wheat	**<u>Nonfood</u>**
Tuna	Wheat Bran	
Turkey	White Rice	Stress
Veal	Whole Grain	Worry
Venison	Wine	Lack of Sleep
Vinegar	Yogurt	

Figure 6.2
Eat less of these foods.

CHAPTER 7

<u>Step Four:</u> Exercise is the Key to Lasting Health

"Take care of your body. It's the only place you have to live."
- Jim Rohn

You weren't thinking about skipping this chapter, were you? I hope not. This is a very important one. In fact, each chapter is equally important in its own way. I'm just kidding with you about skipping it, of course, but my tease emanates from the fact that many people dread the thought of exercising. Our lives are so busy, and it seems that time is moving forward at a much faster pace than it did in the past. You may be saying to yourself; *I don't have time to exercise.* I get it, but the reality is that we make our time. What I mean by this is we have control over what we do with the time we get every day. You have a lot more time available than you think you do.

Before we get into the time-allocating business, let's talk about why exercise is so critical to our overall health. When I say exercise, I'm referring to consistent exercising for five to seven days per week, ideally six or seven days per week. Although any exercise can be helpful, consistent exercise will provide the most beneficial impact on your overall health. If I told you that exercising consistently every week will have anti-inflammatory effects, boost your immune system, reduce infections, and extend your life, would this get your attention? *Yes*, you say. Great, well then, welcome to the club! That was easy. Onto the next chapter!

All kidding aside, exercise has been proven to have many benefits in addition to those listed in the previous paragraph. Here is a list of many of the benefits from frequent exercise:

~ Improves Digestive Function

~ Weight Control

~ Better Sleep

~ Energy Booster

~ Improves Mood

~ Strengthens Immune System

~ Helps Prevent Disease

~ Increases Flexibility and Strength

~ Reduces Stress

~ Boosts Brainpower

~ Optimizes Heart Function

~ Improves Circulation

~ Longer Life

Who would not want to experience all of these fabulous benefits? My purpose for sharing this information with you is to not only eliminate your occurrence of mouths sores, but also increase your overall health. In six months to one year from now, wouldn't it be great for you be free from experiencing mouth sores *and* at the same time be in the best shape of your life? Nothing would make me happier than to know that this was true for you. It would be beautiful music to my ears. I know you thought this book was only going to be about getting rid of those pesky canker sores. Well, it is and it isn't. That's right, we have ourselves a paradox here. If you haven't figured this out by now, you have to be in both great shape and great health in order to be less likely to experience any form of *dis-ease*.

Exercising by itself will not prevent mouth sores. I can attest to this being true. I've exercised my entire adult life and yet I still got chronic mouth sores. I thought I was in great shape and I was likely in pretty good shape. I hardly ever got sick, but I still got mouth sores and, to boot, they got worse over time. In some cases when my immune system was weakened, exercising hard made my mouth sores worse. The important message that I want to convey to you is that I wasn't always doing everything recommended in this book. It was not until I started following every single step that my mouth sores went away for good.

Mouth sores taught me a valuable life lesson when it comes to exercise. I had to learn to listen to my body. You see, I had a tendency to push myself. If I felt tired or run down, I would still go out for my daily run thinking it would make me feel better and more alert. In this respect, I was actually hurting my health. Being someone who has experienced an autoimmune-like disorder, the worst think I could do for my body was to exercise when I was feeling off, run down or overtired. Exercising when the immune system is down is not a good thing to do and can lead to infection and inflammation in the body. Remember the tea pot story? This is where your body is already overflowing and feeling run down and is signally to you that something is off by the way you feel. You then go out and exercise hard for 45 minutes. Now you've really done it by putting your immune system into overdrive which can leads to increased inflammation and illness. That's what would happen to me as there were many times that I manifested mouth sores soon after working out. I kept repeating this same pattern of exercising when I felt off until it dawned on me one day that I might want to start listening to my body. Nowadays, if I ever feel rundown or overtired, I don't exercise that day. It's made a huge difference in my health.

I encourage you to learn how to listen to your body. Be more aware of when you're not feeling one hundred percent. Take it easy. Pamper yourself. Get lots of rest and drink lots of water. Know that rest is the best thing you can do for your immune system when it's off kilter.

Let's get back on track with exercise. It's time for you to get in the time-making business by making exercise a priority in your life. I'm not talking once or twice per week, either. I'm talking five to seven times per week. There are many ways to exercise. The important thing is to get off your duff and start doing something to get your heart rate pumping faster. You don't need to have fancy equipment or belong to a gym. All least not in the beginning. The outdoors can be your gym. Going for a brisk walk is a nice form of exercise. All you have to do is open your front door and start walking.

My favorite form of exercising used to be riding my bike. I love the feeling of coasting on a bike and that feeling like you're flying as you cruise down a hill without pedaling. I used to ride my bike in the spring, summer and fall and then do an elliptical machine during the winter months. I didn't enjoy riding my bike in the winter with the cold air and having to wear a lot of layers. I continued this biking routine for many years until one day I decided to try running. I ran a little during my college years but biking somehow took over as my preferred sport. I assumed that biking would be better for my body. Biking is gentle on the bones and muscles although you can still get a fabulous workout. Biking is a great exercise that almost anyone can do.

You are never too old to start a new form of exercise. After many years of riding my bike, I decided to try running again. I knew from the past that nothing beats running for that euphoric feeling you get after a good run. We've all heard the term "runners high." I wanted to see if I could experience this elevated feeling of joy again. I started running every day. I really started to enjoy it. It didn't take very long for me to experience the runners high. I was hooked!

After a few months, my feet started to hurt a bit and get sore. I tried to ignore it because I was enjoying this form of exercise so much. However, the pain in my feet started to increase. I did a little research online and determined that I had developed plantar fasciitis. Because I kept running a long time with the symptoms, I manifested a serious case of it. I had to get plantar fasciitis night splints to wear while I was sleeping to stretch my tendons. It's a lot of fun going to the bathroom in the dark of the night while trying to walk in those splints. I felt like I was Frankenstein with the way I was teetering as I walked. I was bummed that I had to stop running for a few weeks until my feet got better. After my feet healed, I got back out there and started running again. Six months later, guess what happened? I developed plantar fasciitis again. I had to go through the same healing process and refrain from running for a while.

They say that the definition of insanity is doing the same thing over and over again and expecting a different result. I figured if I started running again without making any changes, I probably had a great chance of becoming the poster boy for plantar fasciitis. I decided to educate myself about this reoccurring issue to find out what I could do about it. I started reading books about proper running technique. I then had the opportunity to hire a professional runner for a few hours to analyze and coach me. I learned how to get into the *chi* of running which is about maximizing performance while eliminating the risk for injury. I learned proper running posture and body motion. I learned how to land on my mid-foot rather than my heal (which was causing the plantar fasciitis by the way.) Those few hours spent with the running coach were the best investment I could ever make for prolonging my running career. I've been running for many years since that coaching session and I have not experienced any foot problems.

So, what's the moral of this story? If you're going to start an exercise you've never done before, make sure that you learn the proper technique. There are tons of free videos online that you can watch that will show you the proper technique for any sport or exercise. Before you start this new activity, watch some videos and know what you're doing. The idea is here is to create better health, not more health problems. Let my experience with running be the nudge for you to make sure you know what you're doing.

Also, depending on the exercise, take time to stretch your muscles and warm up before you start exercising. In the beginning of starting a new exercise, gently ease into it and don't overdo it. Treat your body like the temple that it is. If you are good to your body, it will be good to you. I've had to learn the hard way about this lesson. When I typically ran, my cadence was typically at the same speed. Then I read about the importance of doing both low aerobics and high aerobics. Low aerobics, such as jogging at an easy pace, burns fat. High aerobics, where you're getting your heart rate over 65%, burns glucose. Alternating days of low and high aerobics is really great for the body and keeping you young. By doing this, you are signaling to the brain that you are fit and in the prime of your life. Bodily functions follow the lead of our brain signals and mixing up the pace of exercise improves our overall biology. I started running faster every other day. Things were cranking along fine for a couple of weeks until one day, while running fast up a hill, I tore my calf muscle. I realized that I should have eased into the faster workouts. I also wasn't stretching much before running. This experience taught me the importance of stretching and warming up the muscles. I now exercise and build those leg muscles that I use with yoga, weightlifting or jumping rope.

If you do get an injury, take the time to heal before you get back at it. This was always a hard thing for me to do. I typically needed a doctor to tell me when I could get back to the exercising. When I tore my calf muscle, I didn't go to see a doctor initially because I figured there was nothing they could do about it. I refrained from running for two weeks and then I started up again. I noticed that my calf wasn't fully healed but I wanted to keep running. I purchased some compression bands to wear while walking and running. It was at this time that I broke my pinky toe by slamming it into a leg of the bench in front of our bed. This set me back a couple more weeks. Fortunately, I had made an appointment to see a sports physician right before I broke my toe. This appointment happened a couple of weeks after I broke my toe. When I went to see him, my calf was pretty much all better. He told me that my broken toe saved my calf because, if I would have continued running, I might have re-injured the muscle. It would have not been wise to be running so quickly after injuring that muscle. Hopefully these suggestions are sinking in so you don't have to make the same mistakes. Also, if you ever injure a muscle of any kind, make sure that you massage it frequently after it heals to help reduce any scar tissue.

As I've grown older in calendar years, I've come to see the importance of lifting weights to stay fit and healthy. As we age, we lose both muscle mass and bone mass. Your joints and tendons will start to experience atrophy and the bones and muscles start to decline. This can lead to those wonderful life experiences such as sore joints, aches and pains, and even arthritis. Strength training will drastically slow this decline. Lifting weights a couple of times per week will stop the bone loss, stop the muscle loss and weakening of the tendons and joints. By lifting weights, you'll be signaling to your brain that you are young and fit and in your prime. Be sure to learn proper weightlifting technique. If you can swing it financially, going to a gym is best as they typically have trainers who can show you the proper way to use the equipment. They also typically have the best weightlifting equipment. If you cannot afford the gym, there are exercises you can do at home utilizing items around your house. A quick search online will reveal some books and videos that demonstrate how to do this. My wife and I like to go to the gym as we really like the weight machines. They help ensure proper technique. Take your time with weightlifting and don't overdo it. It's a marathon, not a race. You don't want any injuries to hinder your fitness plan.

My wife and I like to lift weights two times per week. Our gym has some really good classes that combine weightlifting and aerobics. We especially like a form of yoga called body sculpting and we do that twice per week. Go visit all of the gyms in your area to check out their equipment and classes. Gyms are relatively inexpensive these days.

Are you ready to exercise and take up some strength training? I hope so. There are many forms of exercise - running, biking, swimming, hiking, walking, skiing, elliptical, gym classes, etc. Get out there and try some of these activities and mix it up now and then. Stay consistent with it and before long you'll start to feel more energetic, healthy and fit. Your overall immune system will start to improve and, along with all the other steps in this program, you'll be well on your way to eliminating these mouth sores from your life experience.

CHAPTER 8

Step Five: Reduce Stress

*"The greatest weapon against stress is our ability to choose one thought
over another."*
- William James

As you may surmise from your own life experience, stress can play a big role in manifesting mouth sores or any illness and it is worthy of an entire chapter in this book. Depending on what study you look at, stress is the *root cause* for anywhere between 60 and 90% of all illnesses and diseases. Those are some high numbers. Based on my own personal experience and wisdom garnered over the years, I would not say that stress is the root cause of any illness. You have learned about some of the root causes in this book such as Epstein-Barr virus. I would prefer to say stress is the *trigger* for the underlying condition to manifest into *dis-ease* somewhere in your body. Have you ever been really stressed out about something and within a day or two come down with a cold, illness or mouth sore? Most of us would answer this question in the affirmative. Being human means encountering stress during our lives. The important thing is to learn about to cope with the stress.

What causes stress? It's usually happens when we encounter a situation in our life that we perceive to be negative in nature. This encounter subsequently causes all kinds of immediate bodily emotions and reactions which can then lead to increased inflammation and the triggering-of illness or disease. Pause here and go back and read the last three sentences and see if you can find a critical, eye-opening word that can really shift your belief system around stress. Did the word "perceive" stick out in any way? You see, there is really no such thing as negative situations or obstacles. They're only a series of experiences that we encounter throughout our day to day lives. As we encounter each situation or experience, we then consciously or unconsciously react in a way that is either stressful or not. In other words, we are either choosing to label in our mind an experience as negative or positive in nature. This imprint causes the body to manifest either stressful emotions, neutral emotions or happy emotions.

Here's an example of what I mean. Two people can get on a roller coaster side by side. During the roller coaster ride, one of these two people is experiencing joy and euphoria and laughing and screaming in fun. This person's body system is creating a huge spike of endorphins giving them that natural high. Life is good and they are having so much fun. However, the other person sitting beside them, is experiencing extreme fear and high levels of stress. They are screaming and crying in panic because they are so scared at any moment they are going to fall to their death. Their body is in flight or fight mode and their body system is producing cortisol, which increases blood pressure and suppresses the immune system. Same event with two completely opposite reactions going on within their bodies. One is positive and the other is negative. This is a perfect way to demonstrate how the roller coaster ride itself is not stressful. It's our personal reaction to the roller coaster ride that will determine whether it is fun or stressful. This is how it is with everything we experience in life. The more aware you become of this fact, the more opportunity you have to control the amount of stress in your life. I'll discuss some things you can do to help manage and control stress later in this chapter.

Our brain, gut, microbiome and immune system all communicate together. They say our gut is our second brain and, just recently, it was discovered that our microbiome acts like a third brain[8]. We've already talked about how the foods we eat affect our gut, microbiome and immune system. If our brain is also connected to our gut, microbiome and immune system, it only makes sense that emotional stress can impact the same areas. There's a constant back and forth communication going between the brain, gut, microbiome and immune system. They're all interrelated. Emotional stress causes the body to produce chemicals like cortisol when play a role in increasing levels of inflammation. Our gut and microbiome are part of our central nervous system. Stress can affect the gut bacteria in a negative way and prolonged stress can lead to illness and disease. Think of the good bugs in our microbiome as soldiers protecting us by communicating and working with our immune system to shield disorder and disease. If stress causes the microbiome to go haywire, then these soldiers will lose the ability to protect us allowing the enemy (illness) to gain control. We want to protect these soldiers by minimizing the stress we create in our lives.

---

[8] **Ruggiero, Marco. (2017). The Human Microbiota and the Immune System; Reflections on Immortality. Madridge Journal of Immunology. 1. 18-22. 10.18689/mjim-1000106.**

Researchers at Harvard Medical School discovered that meditation or what they called, "the relaxation effect," switched on disease fighting genes in our bodies[9]. They found that people who consistently practiced meditation and relaxation techniques had a significantly greater amount of these disease-fighting genes than people in the control group who did nothing. This study was another confirmation on how our body and state of health is affected by our mood and stress levels. What's even more amazing is, after the study was completed, they had the control group practice relaxation and meditation every day. After two months, they found that their bodies began to change for the better. The genes that fight inflammation and disease and protect the body from illness began to switch on. The bottom line is that the more consistent the practice of meditation and relaxation, the stronger the immune system and likelihood of being free of any kind of bodily disorder.

As I learned more about our body dynamics, I wondered if the gut microbiome and the function of the genes were somehow interconnected. I did some further research and found out that there is a very strong connection between them. A study[10] by researchers at the University of Wisconsin-Madison demonstrated how the microbiome sends signals to the cells to either switch certain genes on or off. This study focused on diet, but it did prove the connection. Based on my own personal experiences and research, I can only surmise that both diet and mindset play a critical role in the health of our microbiome ecosystem. If you're eating a healthy diet while being mentally stressed out for a lengthy period of time,

---

[9] **ncbi.nlm.nih.gov, reference article PMC5961875**
[10] **news.wisc.edu/guts-microbial-community-shown-to-influence-host-gene-expression/**

odds are that you more likely to encounter some sort of health problem. The stress reaction will nullify the effects of healthy eating. Likewise, if you have no stress in your life and you're eating an unhealthy diet for a lengthy period of time, once again, the odds are greater that you might experience illness or disease at some point. The unhealthy diet will supersede the effects of having no stress in your life. Knowing how uncomfortable mouth sores can be, I knew that if I was going to eliminate them for good, I was likely going to have to take a multi-pronged approach. I intuitively knew that no one thing that I could do was going to permanently take care of this chronic problem. I hope this information is helping you to see how important it is to keep stress at a minimum while leading a healthy lifestyle.

When it comes to reducing levels of stress, the best approach is a proactive approach. I've learned the hard way about this. I've actually been involved with personal development since my high school years. It started when my dad gave me a copy of the book, *How to Win Friends and Influence People,* by Dale Carnegie. This book had a profound effect on me and set me on the path of learning how to shape and mold my mind-set. I soon discovered that we actually have a lot of control over the kind of experiences we have. Science has now proven that our thoughts, feelings and beliefs not only affect your health, but they also have a dramatic effect on the circumstances we encounter. Think of our thoughts like antennas that send out signals to the universe of what we want (or don't want) and our feelings like a magnet that draw back to us those experiences that match our thoughts. The fact of the matter is that we are constantly creating our world, consciously or unconsciously, through our thoughts and feelings. Be aware of your thoughts and feelings and learn how to manage them so you can be the captain of your ship of life. I hope by now you are starting to see that the majority of our life experiences are an inside job. I understood this conceptually for many years. However, it wasn't until I experienced a lot of ups and downs in my life, aka that crazy "roller coaster ride of life," that I realized that I needed to do more than read a few positive books.

Our personal growth is a never-ending journey. As I have progressed through mine, I've come to see that spending time improving my mindset is the most important thing I can do on a daily basis. This is where I set the table for my success. It's all about reducing stress and creating positive results with my health and life. When we talked about the importance of physical exercise in the last chapter, I mentioned how important it was to exercise consistently five to seven times per week in order to see positive results with your body. It's just like that with mindset. You have to exercise your mind consistently like you do your body in order to see significant results with your stress levels, your range of positivity, and ultimately your health.

I did not achieve consistent, good results in all areas of my life until I made improving my mindset my number one priority every day. There was a time when I was struggling financially which led to (me manifesting) a lot of stress and some subsequent health scares as a result of it. I knew the importance of a positive mindset, but I wasn't walking the talk as much I could have been doing. Sure, I read many personal development books, attended some workshops and did my best to pay attention to my thoughts and feelings. However, I wasn't as consistent with it. Finally, one day when I was actually thinking about my life and how I was not where I wanted to be with it, I had this spark of inspiration. I realized in that moment that I had to change my priorities and focus if I was every going to see significant, positive change in my life. It was at that point when I decided to make improving my mindset my top priority every day. Now, having never done this before, the thought of meditating every day for the rest of my life seemed a bit daunting. To ease into the task at hand, I committed myself to at least 30 minutes of mindset work every day for 21 straight days. I knew it takes that long to build a new habit so I thought I would commit to 21 straight days and then, after achieving that goal, reevaluate how I felt about it. I was excited to try something different and felt what I was about to do certainly would not harm me in any way. There didn't seem to be much downside to it. So, I spent 30 minutes to an hour per day doing things such as meditating, affirmations, and reading. I would get up a little earlier so I could do this before breakfast. During the first week or two, I remember thinking to myself that *I had to do it* and that I committed myself to doing it, so I needed to honor that commitment. Then a funny thing happened as I approached the 21-day mark. Although the results in my life had not yet changed, I was feeling much better on the inside. I felt more calm and serene. I felt good. I realized something positive was happening to me. As the days and weeks progressed, it went from something that I felt I had to do to something that I *wanted* to do. I started to look forward to what I called my "meditation time" every day. Within a few months, I started to see positive results with my health and finances. I knew I was onto something special here. It was like discovering some ancient secret. It was very powerful! To this day, I make my meditation time my priority every day and I do it before I do anything else.

If you only got from this book that making some "meditation time" for yourself on a daily basis was one of the most important things, if not the most important thing, you can do for yourself, you can drastically improve your life. I have not lost sight of the fact that you want to reduce or eliminate those painful mouth sores. However, from my own personal experience, I know how critical it is to consciously take control of our thoughts, feelings and beliefs. By following this important step, you're going to be learning how to be "at cause" over your life instead of simply reacting to the circumstances you encounter on a daily basis. What you'll really be doing here is learning how to become your *future successful and healthy self right now*. I'm sharing with you the quickest path to get from Point A (your current state of mind and body) to Point B (your future happy, healthy, thriving mind and body.) Can you see it? Can you feel it? Pause here and close your eyes for a few minutes and project yourself out one year from now. Say hello to your future healthy, happy and thriving self. Your future self is in the best shape of their life, hasn't had a mouth sore in months, is at their perfect body weight, is feeling so happy about life and is experiencing success in all areas of their life. Visualize what your future self is doing at this time. What is this version of you thinking? What are you feeling? What beliefs do you carry at this time about yourself? What are you doing on daily basis? What results are you getting in your life? Spend a few minutes basking in the feeling of your future successful self. Then slowly bring your future self back to where you are right now. This is about learning how to *Be* your future successful self *right now*. This is a great exercise to do every night when you're lying in bed before you doze off to sleep. If for some reason it keeps you up, you can do it during your meditation time. If you do this consistently, you'll start to embody your future successful self more and more. You'll start to pay more attention to how you feel and what you think during the day. You'll start to see the connection between your thoughts and feelings and the results you're getting in your life. Everything you're experiencing right now in your life is a reflection of your past thoughts and feelings. The cool thing is that today is the first day of the rest of your life. So is tomorrow and the next day, etc. Every day you get to wake up with a clean slate. You can choose to think good thoughts and feelings throughout that day or bad thoughts and feelings. You can choose to build good habits that day or bad habits that day. You always have a choice and so, as I like to say, *choose wisely.*

I hope this knowledge inspires you to take up some meditation time for the next 21 days to build this incredibly positive habit for yourself. Remember, if you want to have what I have (healthy, happy, thriving body and mind) and what I don't have (mouth sores,) you have to be willing to do everything that I do. You can't cut corners. As your mentor and guide on this journey, I implore you to follow the system, this complete program, as outlined in this book. I promise you that, if you do, you'll become a better person in so many ways. You'll be on top of the mountain ready to take on the world. Your mouth will love you for it and you'll be healthy, happy and fit.

Creating a sacred space for your meditation is a way to solidify your intention for following through with a consistent practice. It will also help you get into the right mood for meditation. I would like to share how you can create a sacred space, literally and mentally, for meditation time. First, I recommend that you choose a specific space in your residence which can be primarily used for mediation time. This could be a cozy corner in your bedroom or any other room. I have an office in my home and in the corner of the office I have a comfy chair and a side table. I have a pole lamp beside the chair. On the walls in the corner I have some pictures that inspire me. On the table, I have things that are important to me. There are objects like gemstones, an angel figure, a candle, a beautiful seashell I found on the beach, a journal, any relevant book I'm reading, and a folder with affirmations and other spiritual writings. It's worth taking the time to gather some things that have a special meaning for you and set up this sacred area for your meditation time.

After your sacred space is set up, you need to think about the time of the day that works best for you. If possible, I recommend that you have your meditation time immediately after you arise in the morning before you do anything else such as eating breakfast. You'll want your mind to be as clear as possible for optimal results. You might have to go to bed a little bit earlier and get up a little earlier in order to make early morning work better. I recommend that you do everything that you can your best to make this meditation time convenient for you. If you are not able to do early mornings, choose the best time where you know you can just relax for 30 minutes or longer without any distractions. Remember, you are committing to doing this for the next 21 days straight. Here is my hard and fast rule I ask you to follow. If you've done it for less than 21 days straight and you skip or forget a day, you'll have to start a new 21-day clock. You have to do this meditation time for 21 straight days before you get to decide if you want to keep doing it. Perhaps having a journal handy will help so you can spend a few minutes every day writing about any positive changes you're noticing with your thoughts, feelings and experiences.

One of the people that inspired me to start meditating every day is Dr. Joe Dispenza[11]. Dr. Joe is a successful author and personal development mentor to the masses. His specialties are neuroscience and neuroplasticity. His focus is about how we can change the neural pathways in our brains to create better habits and results in any area of our lives. Our personalities and beliefs are not hardwired in the brain at birth like science use to think. We can change our personality or habits. It's pretty amazing stuff. Dr. Joe has written several best-selling books and he leads many transformational workshops around the world. I first heard him speak at a conference many years ago right after he published his first book, *Evolve Your Brain*. During his speech, I was shocked when he mentioned that he meditates as much as two hours every day of his life. He further stated that he doesn't get up off his chair until he senses a positive shift with his meditation. I remember thinking to myself, *who has the time to do this?!* Well, fast forward about five years and I found myself reading his second book, *Breaking the Habit of Being Yourself*. (reference). This book took the complex brain science out of his first book and put it into more layman terms. In this remarkable book, Dr. Joe shares his story how he

---

[11] **drjoedispenza.com**

used the technique you learn in the book to overcome a life-threatening accident which caused paralysis. I won't spoil the story. What I like about Dr. Joe is he does a fantastic job of bridging science and spirituality. In fact, he does this better than anyone I know. You'll learn a technique in the last section of the book called Mental Rehearsing. It goes way beyond creative visualization. Looking back to those challenging times, I certainly was at a point in my life where I needed to make some drastic changes. This book and the memory of him sharing how he commits himself daily to meditation inspired me to take the plunge and meditate every single day. It was one of the best decisions I've ever made in my life. To this day, I still practice mental rehearsing every day as part of my meditation time. I recommend that you add all of Dr. Joe's books to your repertoire of reads for improving your life. With *Breaking the Habit of Being Yourself*, there's also an accompanying meditation audio where he leads you through the mental rehearsing technique to help you learn and memorize it. For more information about his books I recommend, the audio, and other resources for meditation, see my website, cankersorecure.com.

Your practice of meditation can be tailored to what's most important to you. I do recommend that you follow some sort of consistent technique to quiet your thoughts and mind. The approach taught by Dr. Joe has parts where you are quieting your mind and other parts where you are guided into certain thoughts and visualizations. This mental rehearsing technique is a great way to begin your journey of reducing stress and changing your mind and body for the better.

Here's another technique for meditation and quieting your mind:

Step 1: Sitting in a comfortable chair with your eyes closed, take a few slow deep breaths in and out. Do this at least 10 times. Next, starting with your attention focused on your feet and then slowly working it up your body to the crown of your head, say the following affirmations taking one deep breath in and out between affirmations: "My feet and ankles are now very relaxed. My shins and calves are now very relaxed. My knees and thighs are now very relaxed. My buttocks, digestive system and genitals are now very relaxed. My lower back, stomach and abdomen are now very relaxed. My upper back and chest are now very relaxed. My neck and face are now very relaxed. The back of my head and crown of my heard are now very relaxed." As you are stating these affirmations, you'll want to actually feel those areas being relaxed. You might start to feel tingles in those areas. The more you practice this, the more you will feel the tingles. Spend some time on each specific area feeling the area becoming very relaxed before you move onto the next area. With practice, you'll learn how to completely relax your body. When you get to the last statement, visualize an energy of light emanating out of the top of your head straight up to infinity. Then, feel yourself receiving positive energy back into your body. Finally, visualize a white light around your body.

Step 2: Let yourself be totally relaxed without thinking any thoughts. Keeping your eyes closed, focus your attention onto your Third Eye. This is the area at the center point of your forehead (above your eyes). The Third Eye is one of your chakras and is associated with enlightenment and mystical insight. It's your connection to your Higher Self and inner wisdom. Simply hold your attention on this area. A way to help you identify this area is to tap it a few times with your finger while your eyes are closed. Simply hold your focus on this area. If you start to have thoughts about something, simply let those thoughts pass through you or, if it helps, visualize those thoughts attached to a hot air balloon that floats away. Don't try to resist them. Just let them float away. Over time, you'll be able to increase the amount of time that you meditate without thinking about things. You'll soon discover how powerful and relaxing meditation can be. Also, if you ever have a personal issue or challenge that you're trying to resolve and you are unsure what to do, you can use this meditation technique to elicit an answer. Simply do these two steps and then, in your mind, ask yourself, "What should I do?" Don't try to think of an answer. Continue to focus on the Third Eye eliminating all thought and patiently wait and see if you get any inspiration. When I do this, sometimes thoughts and answers come to me, not from me. This is how I know that I'm receiving inner wisdom. It's so cool and inspiring when this happens. This wisdom that you get is always the right thing to do, even if it seems counter to what you were thinking, or you don't get the positive results initially from implementing this guidance. This two-step meditation process is a great way to relax and reduce stress in your life. The key is to do it on a regular basis. I urge you to meditate every day.

I cannot emphasize enough the importance of a consistent meditation practice for helping you to reduce your overall stress and improve your health. I believe that my daily practice of meditation by itself has greatly reduced the number of occurrences of mouths sores over the years. I was one of the unfortunate souls who experienced chronic sores. This is because of all of the other reasons you've read about in this book besides stress. Had I not been able to keep my stress levels low, I'm certain I would have experienced them far more than I did. As you've learned, there are many ways to stress our gut microbiome and our immune system. There are many ways that cause inflammation in the body. Stress is one of them. I'm grateful that I had been practicing meditation for many years. It has made an incredible impact in my life, not just with my health. It's also had a positive effect on my finances, my relationships and my mental and emotional state throughout the day. With meditation, there are many things you can add to your practice over time such as affirmations, journaling, expressions of gratitude, and visualization. Allow your practice to grow with you. Have fun with it and honor yourself for making this a priority in your life. Be easy on yourself in the beginning. Don't set high expectations with it. Relax and enjoy strengthening this powerful connection with your higher self.

Before we exit this chapter, there is one other area where we should concentrate on reducing stress: your mouth. This area of your body is the habitat for mouth sores. It's important to be proactive with your mouth as it is with your mind. You want to keep stress at a minimum in your mouth. Good oral hygiene is the key to a healthy mouth. When you brush your teeth, brush carefully. The slightest cuts and scrapes on the gums and inner mouth tissue can be a breeding ground for mouth sores. When you have trauma in the mouth, that area becomes weakened and open to any kind of infection. Brushing your teeth hard can cause problems with your gums and tissue. I use an electric toothbrush which is more accurate and effective in cleaning the teeth. I recommend you use one as well. It will help you prevent trauma on the inside of your mouth. I chuckle at the fact that most people are still brushing their teeth like their ancestors did over 100 years ago. We are creatures of habit, that's for sure. There have been some great improvements with oral care over the years and an electric toothbrush is one of them. If you're not currently using one, I want to encourage you to get with the 21st Century. They are relatively inexpensive now and available almost all retail stores. I've had the same Braun electric toothbrush for at least ten years. I highly recommend this brand. Be sure to replace your toothbrush heads on a frequent basis. Also, be sure to use toothpaste that does not contain Sodium Laurel Sulfate (SLS) as it has been known to trigger mouth sores.

I have a habit of biting my cheeks when I eat. This motivated me to chew more slowly. My inner cheek tissue is really close to my teeth and so this used to happen to me frequently. Whenever this happens, I dab some myrrh on there right away and it will reduce the swelling immediately. Chewing slowly is also good for your digestive system. Make it a point to start chewing your food more slowly. This will help you prevent biting your cheeks. I want to reiterate that any trauma to the mouth can be fertile ground for mouth sores. Finally, make sure that you floss daily and the more times per day, the better. Flossing is critical for good oral health. I floss after every meal if possible. Flossing helps prevent tartar, bacteria, inflammation and disease.

Reducing stress in both your mind and body is not a passive process. It starts with assessing where you are and where you want to be. Your mind and body are great barometers if you listen to them. Take some time to do an honest assessment of your health and stress levels. Rate yourself on a scale of one to ten with ten being perfect. Be honest with yourself. Decide right now that you want to be a ten in mind and body. There's no reason you can't get close. It's a journey. I'll be striving to get to ten in mind and body for the rest of my life. I'm passionate about health and well-being and becoming the best person that I can possibly be. If you feel like this is a big stretch for you, it's okay. If you are really sick or chronically ill, don't fret. All you need to do assess your current situation and then create a plan to better it. And be sure to follow through on your plan. There are many good ideas in this book. Baby steps are good. I have a question for you. Can you jump ahead farther from starting from a standstill or taking two backwards and then using the momentum from starting a couple of steps behind that starting spot to leap forward? If you take those two steps back first, you then gain some forward momentum with your body and end up further than you would from starting from a standstill. Take those steps back to assess yourself and then plan your journey ahead. This will give you some extra momentum for healing yourself.

Your life will improve immensely when you learn to be the captain of your ship of life. It's about knowing where you are, where you want to go, and the steps you need to take to get there. This process will help you go from reacting to your world to being *at cause* over your life. This is the only way to become the best person that you can possibly be. I acknowledge you getting this far in the book. It shows that you really want the best for yourself, that you desire to heal your body and mind.

CHAPTER 9

Twenty-five Healthy Habits

"Your outcomes are a lagging measure of your habits."
- James Clear

I'm excited to share with you twenty-five healthy habits that you can perform on a consistent basis to reduce stress, better your health, keep those stinky mouth sores at bay, and ensure that you live a long and productive life. These tasks do not take much extra effort and can easily be integrated into your daily/weekly routine. They are little minor adjustments that you can do that will make a huge and positive impact. One of my favorite sayings is, *focus on the little things because the little things are the big things.* I truly believe that these minor tweaks to your way of going about your day can make all the difference in your quality of life. Some of the recommendations in this chapter have already been previously discussed. I have added them here to reinforce the message and give you a bookmark for some great daily habits.

If you would like to go for the gusto, feel free to immediately add all or most of them to your daily and weekly routine. If it seems a bit overwhelming to do many at once, perhaps start with one or two recommendations and do them for a few days to a week. Then, add another one or two of the suggestions every few days. Keep repeating this process until you are doing all of the recommendations listed in this chapter. Have fun with it and give yourself a pat on the back for following through and being consistent with integrating the list. You'll start to feel happier and healthier before you know it. When you feel good, good things happen to you. Treat your body like the temple it is and it will reward you in kind.

A key thought to remember is, *you get what you expect out of life.* Expect great health and great health will happen for you. Let me share one of my favorite stories with you to emphasize this point: one day, a farmer was tending to his crops by the side of the road. A car comes to a stop beside the farmer. The farmer sees a family of four inside the car. The husband rolls down his window and says, "Howdy there, sir. We are thinking about moving to your town and we're wondering what the people are like here?" The farmer paused and looked down for a second and then responded, 'What are the folks like in your current town?" The man replied, "Where we come from, the people are very conniving and will take the shirt off your back if you are not careful. They're not kind at all. That's why we're moving." The farmer replied, "Well, you'll find the people of our town are just like that!" The man thanked the farmer and said they would check out the next town. Later that day, the same farmer was tending his crops and another car came to a stop on the road beside him. The man got out of his car and said, "Hello there. May we have a minute?" The farmer said "Sure, how can I help you?" The man said, "We are thinking about putting our roots down here in your town and we wanted to know what the town folk are like here?". The farmer replied, " What are the town folk like where you come from?" The man replied, "Sir, where we come from, the people are so nice and friendly, and they would do anything for you. They are very kind people and we love them and will miss them dearly." The farmer replied, "Well, I am happy to tell you that you will find the people in our town are exactly like the people of your town." The man replied, "Wonderful. This will likely be our new home!". The moral of this story and what this wise farmer knew is that the world responds in kind to you. Express hate and meanness to the others, and you'll experience a lot of hate and meanness from others coming back into your life. If you come from the heart and express love and kindness to others, then you'll receive a lot of love and kindness from those around you.

Let's now get to the list so you can start building some wonderful new habits for yourself. As you follow these recommendations, know and believe that by doing them consistently, you will experience some amazing positive results. Have the attitude that you will see it when you believe it rather than you'll believe it when you see it.

Drink a Big Glass of Water First Thing in the Morning

We spent an entire chapter coving the subject of water. You will want to be mindful of how much water you drink every day. The most important time for drinking water is as soon as you wake up in the morning before you do anything else. Your body is dehydrated after going seven to eight hours without water. It is so important to replenish and rehydrate it as soon as you can. When you leave your bedroom, go straight to the kitchen and get yourself a very large glass of purified or good spring water. I recommend at least 20 to 24 ounces. Drink your first glass of water within 15 minutes and be sure to drink plenty of water throughout the day as outlined in Chapter 5.

Drink Celery Juice 30 Minutes After Finishing First Glass of Water

Wait at least 30 minutes after drinking your first glass of water for the day, then drink 16 ounces of celery juice. Celery juice is a superfood that will kill viruses and remove toxins from your body. It is the number one thing you can do to kill off the Epstein-Barr virus. It's worth investing in a good juicer. One celery stalk or bag of celery will typically produce 16 ounces of celery juice. Use organic celery if possible and rinse it off good before putting it into the juicer. Wait at least 30 minutes to one hour after you drink the celery juice before eating breakfast.

Meditate Every Day

Create a sacred space as your place to meditate every day. This is the best habit you can create to reduce the level of stress in your life. It will also help you become more present and aware. If possible, the first thing in the morning is the best time to meditate because your mind is very clear. As soon as I grab my glass of water, I head to my sacred space for my meditation time. Refer back to Chapter 8 for suggestions on how to do this properly. I recommend at least 30 minutes of meditation time per day. Do as much as you can. Commit to at least 21 straight days and then see how you feel. If you miss a day, start the 21-day commitment period over again.

Wash Your Hands Upon Entering Your Home

This one tip could really save you from having many illnesses over your lifetime. Create the great habit of washing your hands as soon as you walk into your home after being out and about. You may need to create some reminder for yourself initially. You could put a sticky note on your door where you will clearly see it. Move the sticky note around frequently so you don't get used to it being in the same place, otherwise you may not be aware of it after a while. Keep some sort of reminder until this becomes second nature for you. When you are out and about, be conscious of not touching your face. Keep a hand sanitizer in your car and use each time you get into the car. Wash your hands before every meal to keep germs off your food.

Exercise At Least Five Days Per Week

As we discussed in Chapter 7, consistent exercise is very important to your overall health. In order to be able call yourself an athlete, you have to be one who exercises consistently and frequently, at least five days per week. This habit will keep you in good shape and improve your overall health. It will aid in preventing *dis-ease*. In order for you to become ultra-healthy, you have to make exercising a priority in your life. If you work during weekdays, in addition to Saturday and Sunday, you only have to find at least 3 workout times during the work week. Surely you can find 45 minutes before work, during your lunchtime or after work. You can do this!

Lift Weights

As we age, we lose muscle mass. When this happens, the body is signaling the brain that we are getting older and to let the normal cycles of atrophy happen to us. Lifting weights builds muscle mass, strengthens and tones our bodies and makes us look and feel good. Most importantly, we are signaling to the brain that we are still youthful resulting in a slowdown of the atrophy process. Exercising and weightlifting is a powerful combination for keeping you young and healthy. If you have access to a gym, great. If not, you can get some inexpensive dumbbells or elastic bands to use at home. You only have to lift weights twice per week in order to call yourself a weightlifter too!

Do Yoga or Stretching Habitually

Along the same lines of exercising and weightlifting, stretching is another good way to maintaining your health and youthful image. Keeping your body limber is good for your overall health. Take some yoga classes. There are hundreds and hundreds of free yoga and stretching classes online that you can do from the comfort of your home. There is no excuse to not do this. I highly recommend yoga because is a powerful way to improve health, flexibility, balance and strength. Make sure you learn the correct way to do the poses to prevent injury. And, you only have to do yoga at least twice per week to call yourself a yogi! If you don't want to do yoga, there are many helpful stretches that you can do for 15 or 20 minutes every day or two. A simple search online will yield you many good ideas.

Practice Gratitude

This is a great thing to do during your mediation time. Gratitude is probably the next greatest energy besides love. In order to have more of what you like and desire in your life, it is important to be grateful for what you already have. On a daily basis, write down or state out loud at least ten things you are grateful for. See what new things you can come up with every day. Feel the emotion of gratitude when you say these ten things. Don't just say them quickly. Feel and express the emotion of gratitude. Take this a step further and make it point to express gratitude throughout your day. Gratitude is a great attraction energy. Lots of great things will happen for you when you emanate gratitude. One of the things I do is set my phone alarm to go off at 9 am, 3 pm, and 9 pm. When this happens, I check in with myself to see where my thoughts are, and I take a minute to feel gratitude for some things. This has done wonders for me!

Pay Yourself 10% First

What's this have to do with this book about health? Well, having to deal with finances or lack thereof is one of the leading causes of stress in our society. Why not nip this one in the bud immediately? I wish I had started doing this when I was much younger. Here's how it goes: anytime you have any kind of income or money coming to you, take ten percent right off the top and put into a savings/investment fund. Do this before you pay bills or use the money for anything else. You won't even notice it missing. It will be easy to do. You'll be amazed at how fast this fund grows. You'll also be alleviating some serious stress in the future.

Stretch for Five Minutes Before Getting Out of Bed in the Morning

This is an easy and simple way to stay limber as you are slowly becoming more alert. Right after waking up and while still laying in the bed, do a little stretching. Do each of these stretches to a 20-second count. Bring your knees up to your chest. Then, with one leg straight and one leg bent, cross the bent knee over the straight leg. Then switch and do the other leg. Next, with one leg bent and foot planted on the bed, cross the other leg's foot on top of the knee, put both hands on the shin and pull forward to stretch the thigh. Then switch sides. Next, bring your feet together and allow your legs to fall to the side to make a diamond shape. While the legs are wide open, take your one arm in straight line over your chest and use the other arm to wrap around it above the elbow and pull the straight arm further into your chest for a shoulder stretch. While maintaining the same pose with the legs, do the other arm. You can add your own stretches to the mix. Important: when you are ready to get out of bed, turn and lay on your side facing out, and push yourself up with your arms. Don't try to solely use only your back muscles to get up. Let your arms do the pushing. This is going to save you a back injury or two during your lifetime.

Limit Liquids Around Meals

Don't drink anything within 15 minutes prior to or within one hour after a meal to allow your digestive enzymes to work properly. Eating healthy is critical but also giving the body space to digest the food properly is just as important. Limiting fluids during meals helps the body to better breakdown the food and absorb the nutrients. If you drink a lot of liquid with a meal, it will also slow down the emptying of the stomach which can result in you becoming bloated.

Don't Sit or Stand for Long Periods of Time

Here's a little secret that can help you optimize your health and live a long and productive life: don't sit for hours at a time and don't stand for hours at a time. Mix it up as much as possible. Sitting for long periods of times is not good for your health and reduces the effects of all that exercising that you do. It can lead to weight gain and other health problems. Standing for long periods of time can negatively impact your circulation and lead to cardiovascular disease. If you typically sit or stand for long periods of time, make a point to do the opposite many times during the day. If your work requires you to do one or the other for long periods of times, you can always find a way to mix it up, even for a brief moment. Even doing this for minute or two periodically will benefit you. I have a laptop stand by my desk. I find myself doing 15 to 20-minute intervals of sitting and standing. I've trained my body to tell me when it's time to make the change.

Become a Truth Seeker

The path to fully optimizing your life is obtained by building both your inner and outer awareness. When you understand the world within in you and world outside of you, you are better able to make the right choices and decisions for achieving best results. You build your inner awareness by doing things like meditation, reading and learning about the mind-body connection, and following and trusting your intuition. You build your outer awareness by learning what's really going on in the world around you. You do this by seeking and finding sources of information that have a track record of being truthful. You may have to dig deep to find these sources. There is much propaganda in our world today. Remember, nothing is true unless you determine it is so.

Avoid Refined Sugar

Refined sugar is a poison and toxin to your body. It feeds the unhealthy viruses, bacteria and fungus in your body. Over time, this can lead to an array of health problems such as diabetes, heart disease, liver disease, and cancer. When your liver is affected in a harmful way, it can lead to all kinds of health problems in your body including mouth sores. Use alternative natural sweeteners such as coconut sugar, honey, maple syrup, stevia, monk fruit, dates (on salads and in smoothies,) and xylitol. Also be sure to avoid high fructose corn syrup as it is just as bad as refined sugar. Eliminating these toxins from your body is one of the best things you can do for your health.

Use Sunscreen

Most of us are already aware of the harmful effects of the rays of our sun and yet we don't use sunscreen as frequently as we should. If you are going to be out in the sun for more than 15 minutes at a time, put some sunscreen on your exposed areas first. Use a sunscreen with at least a 30 SPF protection. The higher, the better. It's worth buying the highest quality and most natural sunscreen you can find to reduce toxins on your skin. A side benefit to using sunscreen consistently is that your skin will age well, and you will be reducing the amount of age spots on your face, arms and hands.

Take Supplements

It is a well-known fact that the soil in our ground does have the level of nutrients that is used to have. Many generations of farming prioritized productivity over care of the topsoil. This resulted in the soil losing many important nutrients that would typically get absorbed into foods that are grown. It is important to supplement our bodies with a really good multivitamin to make up for the loss of nutrients in our food. Review Chapter 6 for specific supplement recommendations for dealing with your mouth sores.

Eat Organic and Non-GMO foods

A wonderful byproduct of following the protocols in this book is the elimination of viruses and toxins in your body. While this is happening, you don't want to be ingesting new poisons and toxins. Non-organic food contains many pesticides which are toxic to your body. Although the media pushes the narrative that GMO foods are safe, there are many studies to contradict this message. You are what you eat. This reminds me of the comical scene of a guy with the hole in his rowboat. Instead of plugging the hole, he frantically scooping out the water and eventually he and his boat sinks. We have to plug the hole of toxins by not eating foods that contain them. Also, if you eat meat and/or fish, eat only organic, grass-fed meat and/or wild caught fish. Avoid eating fish that contains high levels of mercury such as tuna and swordfish.

Self-Reflect, Assess Your Life Regularly

At least once per week or every two weeks, take some time to assess where you are and what you have accomplished and achieved since the last time you did this exercise. Review your personal health as well as your life goals and dreams. Review your notes from your last assessment session. Create a to-do list for the coming week(s). If you have a loved one, perhaps do this exercise together. My wife and I like to go to a coffee shop every two weeks and do this together. We share our personal goals and discuss the goals and dreams we want to achieve together. You'll find that regularly assessing your life will help catapult you to where you ultimately want to be. It is also very important to write down your goals. Studies show that writing out your goals greatly increases the likelihood that you will achieve them. I always like to say, *"If you don't know where you're going, you'll always be on the road to nowhere."*

Use a Simple and Effective To-Do List

In the early 1900's, Charles Schwab, President of Bethlehem Steel, asked a successful business consultant, Ivy Lee, to help him increase the productivity of his company. Lee said he would do it and after three months, suggested that Schwab could pay him for whatever the value he received. Lee then instructed each of his Schwab's executives to, at the end of each day, write down the six most important things they need to accomplish the next day. They were to prioritize these six things in order of importance. The next day they were to focus only on the most important task and only move on to the next one after completing the first one. Same for the remaining tasks. At the end of the day, they were to move any unaccomplished tasks to the next day's list and repeat the same process the following day. These instructions increased company productivity so well that, after three months, Schwab gave Lee a check for $25,000, which is the equivalent of over $430,000 in today's money. I have used this simple to-do list for many years can attest that it works great!

Chew Slowly and Eat in Moderation

I have to admit this was a tough one for me. I come from a family of fast eaters. This took me a long time to see the value in it. There is no excuse to not do this and it might help to understand why you should. Chewing slower greatly aids your digestion by allowing your body to produce more digestive juices. It will also prevent you from gaining any unnecessary weight because you will feel full quicker. Lastly, it will help you eat more moderately and enjoy your food. Doing so will help to reduce stress in both your mind and body. The easiest way to achieve this is to take a bite of food and then immediately put your fork down on the plate. Chew each bite of food into the tiniest of pieces before swallowing. Do not pick up your fork again until you have slowly chewed and then swallowed that particular bite of food. While you're at it, if you're with someone, add some conversation between bites. Savor each bite of food and make eating an experience to enjoy.

Become a Fast Flosser

What I am really conveying here is to floss after every meal if possible. You might be thinking, *"Are you nuts?"* I did say *if possible*. When you're home, floss after every meal. If you can floss at your work after a meal, then do it. If not, that's okay. I don't think I need to spend too much time discussing the benefits of flossing. Everyone knows that frequent flossing helps prevent tooth decay and gum disease. The neat thing is that the more you floss, the easier and quicker it gets. For me, flossing is now just like brushing my teeth. I can floss my entire mouth in a minute or two because I've done it so many times. I challenge you to become a fast flosser. You up for the task? Your mouth and teeth will thank you for it.

So will your pocketbook in the long run. We all know how high those dental bills can be.

Focus on Solutions, Not Problems

In Chapter 8, we discussed how there is no such thing as obstacles. There are only experiences that we have where we perceive them to be obstacles. We make them obstacles in our mind. Knowing this makes it much easier to solve our problems. If the *problem* was created in our mind, then so too can the solution be created in our mind. Don't dwell on the negative aspects of the issue at hand but rather accept it for what it is in that moment. Have the attitude that there is always a blessing to be found with every perceived obstacle (that you create in your mind from the experience you are having.) Place all of your energy and effort into finding or creating potential solutions. A key strategy when encountering an *obstacle* is to pay attention to your thoughts. Keep your mind focused on solutions. If you're stuck, affirmations can help. I would like to share my all-time favorite affirmation that my wife and I created together. This is about letting go and letting God: "Divine Order is now manifesting in this situation, creating the best possible outcome for me." Say this over and over again, especially when those negative thoughts start to creep in. In won't be long before you internalize the meaning of it and feel the truth of it. The perfect solution will then happen for you. It always has for me!

Find a Passion

If your work is your passion, you are one of the few and fortunate ones. We are conditioned to believe that if we find our passion, the money and freedom will soon follow. This could not be further from the truth. The majority of people have a passion that is a hobby of theirs. Some make some money from it, some don't. Some do it for the pure pleasure of following their bliss. Finding a passion will reduce stress and keep you happy and fulfilled with life. Remember, the body reacts to our emotions. Keep your emotions happy and your body will follow suit. Find something to do that rocks your boat. The more the passions, the more the merrier you shall be.

Get a Good Night's Sleep

In order for our bodies to function properly in the long term, it is important that we get sufficient sleep. Most people need 7-8 hours of sleep per night to maintain their health and perform at optimal levels. Sleep can be a challenge for many people. Here are some tips if you're having some sleep issues: try going to bed as soon as you get that tired feeling at night. Then, set your alarm to wake up at the same time every day. If it's hard to settle down at night, try reading a good book or writing out your thoughts and the things that are occupying your mind. Don't drink many fluids after 7 pm at night. This will prevent you from having frequent visits to the bathroom during the middle of the night which interrupt your sleep. There are many suggestions out there for how to get a good night's sleep. Do a little research and try different things. Look to create a routine that works on a consistent basis.

Practice Mindfulness

Mindfulness is about being present and becoming aware of your thoughts. Meditating every day will increase your mindfulness quotient. When you do meditate, set an intention for the day to be fully aware of your thoughts. Or, do this before you get out of bed every morning. Affirm, "Throughout my day today, I will be fully aware of my thoughts and I will think only good thoughts." A helpful tip, similar to what I shared in the Gratitude section, is to set the alarm on your phone to go off every hour or two throughout the day. When this happens, take a mini meditation for a couple of minutes. Close your eyes and breathe deeply. Stay present with your breath. If your mind starts to wander or have thoughts, bring yourself back to the present moment by imagining them floating away on a hot air balloon. Practice being present with yourself and with others. Become a good listener and you will become more mindful. Increasing your mindfulness quotient will reduce stress and improve your health and life.

CHAPTER 10

The New You

"Beautiful are those whose brokenness gives birth to transformation and wisdom."
- John Mark Green

Congratulations are in order! You have made it this far in the book. You have stuck with it and now you know everything that you can do to rid yourself of these painful mouth sores. You are to be acknowledged for caring enough about yourself and your health to want to make positive changes. You are now ready to create that New You.

You may have already started implementing many of these suggestions while reading through each chapter. I know I would be doing this if I was having to live through painful mouth sores again. May I suggest that you go back and read everything again and create a to-do list for each chapter. Then start knocking off those items one by one with the highest priority items listed first (following the healthy habit suggestion of using to-do lists.)

Here is a very important question I would like you to answer right now: are you willing to do everything suggested in this book? If your answer is yes, great. If your answer is no, why not? Isn't your health more important than everything else in your life? Remember what it feels like to have the excruciating pain and discomfort from a large mouth sore? Do you want to keep experiencing them or do you want the satisfaction that comes from conquering them once and for all? Do you want to live a long, healthy and productive life or do want to continue having health issues? If you need to spend time contemplating this, that's okay. As your mentor on this short journey, I believe in you and I know you can do it!

What I have shared with you in this book is what I absolutely know works for me. I only know what works for me. I can vouch for everything contained within these pages because I've done all of it. If you're not willing to follow all of the suggestions in this book and you're still experiencing mouths sores, then you'll know why. You have to be willing to do everything. Also, it's very important to give yourself at least six months to experience significant results. It may take longer. Be patient with yourself and allow your body to change for the better. It is possible that you might have some detox effects from changing your diet and following this protocol. If that happens, be okay with it and know that it is helping you be healthier in the long run. Remember, sometimes you have to take a couple of steps backwards in order to take a giant leap forward.

This book is giving you a process to speed up from getting from point A, where you are right now, to point B, your future healthy and happy self. The quickest way to become your future healthy and happy self is to *Be* that person right now. By taking action and doing everything outlined in this book, you will be living your future healthy and happy life right now, as if you were symptom-free and healthy. Would not a healthy, symptom-free person be doing everything recommended within these pages? When you *Be* the person you expect to be six months to one year from now, and you *Do* what this person would be doing with your actions, you will *Have* what that person will have much faster than any other process. *Be, Do, Have. Be* the person you want to be, *Do* what that person would do, and then you'll *Have* what that person would have.

When you have had no or very rare experiences of mouth sores for at least six months, feel free to reintroduce some of the foods that are known to cause mouth sores. Do it slowly and carefully and only reintroduce one food at a time. Don't eat too much of that one food right away. Take it slow. I have found that I can pretty much eat anything now although I still avoid spicy and peppery foods as I just don't think they are good for my body type. If you get a mouth sore after reintroducing a certain food, avoid eating it. Perhaps you can try again in a few months.

If you are still getting a mouth sore on occasion, don't give up. Give it more time. If this happens, you are likely only going to get one rather than multiple ones at once. They will usually be smaller, and they will clear up much faster. Remember to become more aware of your mouth. If you ever feel any tingle or soreness, don't take a chance. Don't wait to find out if it becomes a mouth sore. Get some of your myrrh and dab it on the spot right away. It will likely dissipate very quickly.

Remember, there is also a full list of all of the recommended resources from this book on my website, cankersorecure.com, which you can access at any time. This gives you a convenient starting place to get whatever products you would like to have. If you have found the information in this book to be helpful and if it has impacted you in a positive way after a period of time, I would love to hear your story. Feel free to share your story with me. There will be a way to contact me on my website.

Finally, give thanks to those pesky mouth sores. There is always a blessing in every *perceived* obstacle. You just have to look for it. If you have implemented all of the ideas and suggestions in this book then, in addition to reducing or eliminating mouth sores, you are becoming healthier than you have ever been during your entire life. This is cause for much gratitude and celebration!

Thank you for allowing me to be your guide throughout this process. I wish you great health and much happiness in the days ahead.